Self-as

# Pe                                                                    y

## H Donald Glenwright
**BDS, MDS, FDS, RCS (Eng)**

**Head of Unit of Periodontology**
University of Birmingham
School of Dentistry
Birmingham
England

**Director**
Birmingham Dental Hospital
School of Dental Hygiene
Birmingham
England

## J Dermot Strahan
**BDS, MGDS, FDS, RCS (Eng)**

**Head of Department of Periodontology**
Institute of Dental Surgery
Eastman Dental Hospital
London
England

**Director**
Eastman Dental Hospital
School of Dental Hygiene
London
England

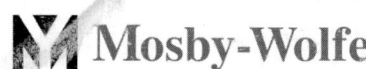 Mosby-Wolfe

London · Baltimore · Barcelona · Bogotá · Boston
Buenos Aires · Carlsbad, CA · Chicago · Madrid
Mexico City · Milan · Naples, FL · New York
Philadelphia · St Louis · Seoul · Singapore
Sydney · Taipei · Tokyo · Toronto · Wiesbaden

**Related titles published in Mosby's Testing series include:**

Dental Technology
Endodontics
Operative Dentistry
Oral Anatomy, Embryology and Histology
Oral Medicine
Oral Radiology
Paediatric Dentistry
Paedodontics
Prosthodontics

Production:          **Cathy Martin**

Cover Design:        **Lara Last**

Publisher:           **Geoff Greenwood**

# Preface

This book is designed for use by all those who wish to test and update their knowledge of modern periodontology. We hope that it will prove helpful to dental students and student hygienists, as well as to qualified members of both professions, as part of continuing education. It will be especially useful to those who are studying for higher qualifications.

The questions, which have been randomised to maintain the reader's interest, have been given comprehensive answers and have been chosen to cover the whole range of periodontology and related areas. They have been set by contributors who are all acknowledged experts in their field.

It should be noted that, for convenience of reference, each question has been allocated its own number and that each figure takes its number from the question it illustrates. As some questions are not illustrated, figure numbers do not always run consecutively.

# Acknowledgements

We are grateful to all the contributors who worked so carefully, setting the questions and preparing the answers for this book. Much more work was involved than any of us expected.

The secretarial and word-processing skills of April Cook, Katie Glenwright, Marie Jones, Teresa Kelly and Karen Lim Ah Ken are gratefully acknowledged, as is the help so willingly given by Mike Sharland and Marina Tipton of the Photographic Unit, University of Birmingham School of Dentistry.

We thank Dr Raman Bedi, Dr Stephen Flint, Mr John Hamburger, Mr Peter Hull, Mr John Morris, Dr Paul O'Reilly and Dr Peter Rock for allowing us to use their photographic material.

Figures 47 and 86 are reproduced by kind permission of the Editor of the *Journal of Clinical Periodontology*, and Figure 98 by that of the Editor of *Dental Update*.

Finally, our thanks must go to our wives, who endured many evenings without conversation during the preparation of this book.

# Dedication

To our wives, Gill and Anne.

# List of contributors

**Professor Martin Addy,** BDS, MSc, PhD, FDS RCS (Eng). Professor of Periodontology, University of Bristol.

**Dr Iain LC Chapple,** BDS (N'cle), PhD (B'ham), FDS RCPS (Glas). Senior Lecturer in Restorative Dentistry (Periodontology), University of Birmingham School of Dentistry.

**Associate Professor Noel Claffey,** BDS, MA, MDentSc, FDS RCPS (Glas). Head of Periodontal Unit, Chairman of Postgraduate Studies, The Dental School, Dublin.

**Professor Jeremy M Hardie,** BDS, PhD, Dip Bact, FRC Path. Professor and Head of Department of Oral Microbiology, The London Hospital Medical College, Dental School.

**Mr David G Hillam,** BDS (Durham), MDS (N'cle), FDS RCS (Eng). Consultant in Restorative Dentistry, Liverpool University Dental Hospital. Director, Liverpool School of Dental Hygiene. Honorary Lecturer in Clinical Dental Surgery, University of Liverpool.

**Dr Michael Saxby,** DDS, FDS RCS (Ed). Senior Lecturer and Honorary Consultant, University of Birmingham School of Dentistry.

**Professor Robin A Seymour,** PhD, FDS RCS (Ed). Professor of Restorative Dentistry, Department of Restorative Dentistry, The Dental School, Newcastle-upon-Tyne.

**Dr M Jeremy Shaw,** BDS (Lond), DDS (B'ham),FDS RCS (Eng), MRD. Consultant in Restorative Dentistry, Honorary Senior Lecturer, University of Birmingham School of Dentistry.

**Dr Linda Shaw,** BDS Hons, PhD, FDS RCS (Eng), LDS RCS. Senior Lecturer and Consultant in Paediatric Dentistry, University of Birmingham School of Dentistry and Birmingham Children's Hospital.

**Mr David G Smith,** BDS, DRD, FDS RCS (Ed). Consultant in Restorative Dentistry. Consultant in Administrative Charge of Periodontal Department, Newcastle-upon-Tyne Dental Hospital. Director, Newcastle School of Dental Hygiene.

**Professor Trevor F Walsh,** DDS (B'ham), MSc (Lond), BDS (Lond), FDS RCS (Eng). Senior Lecturer and Consultant in Restorative Dentistry, Charles Clifford Dental Hospital, Sheffield.

**1** This 21-year-old male patient was referred by his dentist to a dental hygienist for scaling, polishing and instruction in oral hygiene. Two days after this had been done he returned with this painful ulcer at the gingival margin of 43. There was an identical lesion associated with 33. The dentist referred the patient to hospital, fearing he might have a blood dyscrasia. What is the likely cause of this lesion?

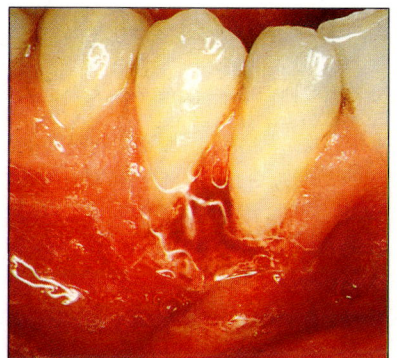

**1**

**2** This 19-year-old final year student (**2A**) presented in the month of June, with gingival pain and ulceration of 1 week's duration. He was a non-smoker, had good oral hygiene and there was no evidence of trauma. A diagnosis of acute necrotising ulcerative gingivitis (ANUG) was made, oral hygiene instruction (OHI) given and prophylaxis performed. He was prescribed metronidazole 200 mg t.d.s. for 5 days, chlorhexidine 0.2% mouthwash, twice daily, and reviewed 10 days later. At review the lesions had deteriorated.
(a) What are the possible reasons for this?
(b) How should the patient be managed at this stage?

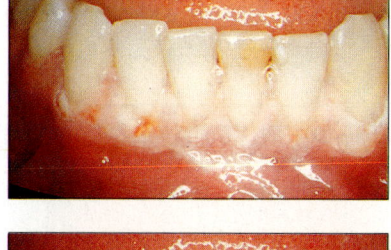

**2A**

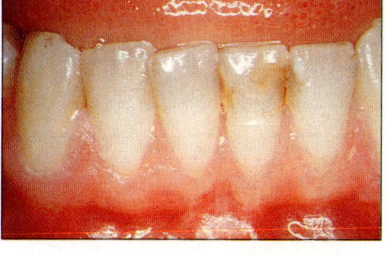

**2B**

**3** In some patients, including both children and adults, aggressive forms of periodontal disease are observed which result in rapid progression and loss of supporting structures of the teeth. A variety of names has been used to describe such conditions, including localised juvenile periodontitis (LJP) and rapidly progressive periodontitis (RPP).
(a) Which micro-organisms have been specifically associated with LJP?
(b) Which antibiotic is sometimes prescribed to treat patients with LJP?
(c) Which micro-organisms are thought to be associated with RPP?
(d) Are there any known virulence factors produced by micro-organisms associated with LJP or RPP?

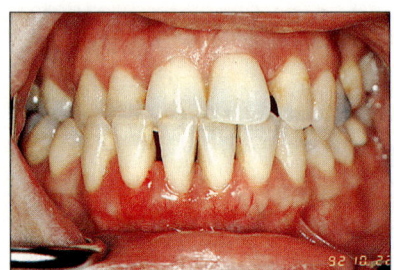 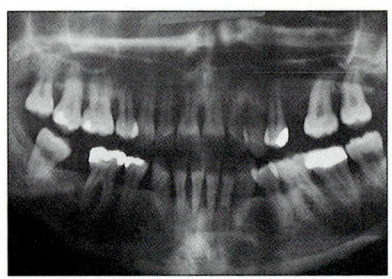

**4** This 28-year-old female patient is complaining of bouts of gingival bleeding and loosening of teeth. On examination the gingivae appear slightly inflamed. Her radiograph is shown in **4B**.
(a) Indicate your likely diagnosis.
(b) Is there any pattern this disease may follow?
(c) What treatment is indicated?

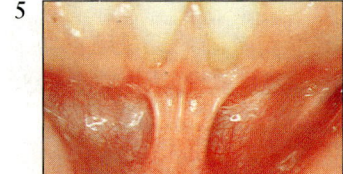

**5** This photograph shows a patient with a high fraenal attachment and shallow sulcus in the lower anterior region. What implications do these anatomical features have for oral hygiene and what can be done to correct the features of this area of the mouth?

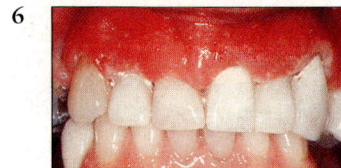

**6** This patient recently had a temporary crown fitted to 23. Two days later, he complained of soreness and a burning sensation in the adjacent gingival tissues. What is the most likely cause and how would you manage the case?

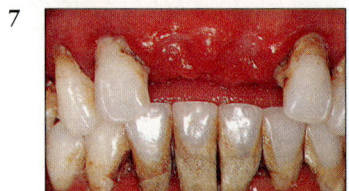

**7** This patient suffers from diabetes mellitus. Does this photograph show any features which are pathognomonic of the condition?

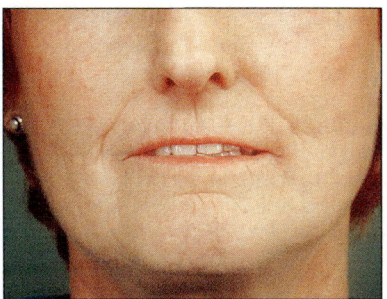
8A

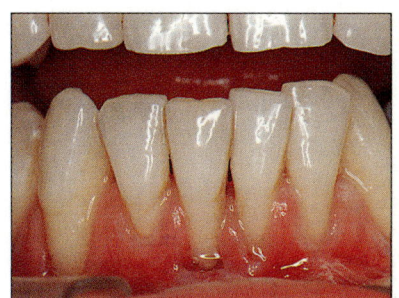
8B

**8** This 52-year-old female patient has a connective tissue disorder, two of the oral manifestations of which are seen in **8A** and **8B**. Her hands are shown in **8C**.
(a) What signs can be seen and what is the condition?
(b) What oral and periodontal changes occur in this disease?
(c) How should such patients be maintained?

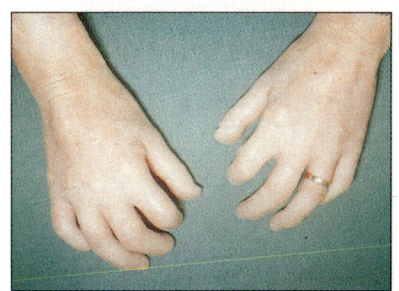
8C

**9** This 25-year-old woman presented complaining of some discomfort from the palatal aspect of her upper anterior teeth. Examination revealed that she had experienced recession of the gingiva palatal to the upper incisors. The overbite was complete, the gingival sulcus depth less than 3mm and there was some evidence of tooth wear.
(a) What is the diagnosis?
(b) How should the patient be treated?

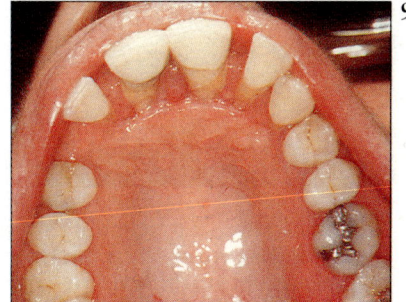
9

**10** What are the causes of immunodeficiency and how can they affect the periodontium?

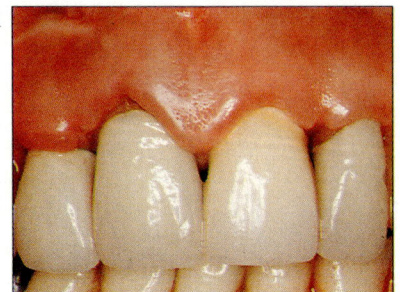

**11** This 50-year-old female is a heavy smoker and has gingival recession and recurrent soreness in the maxillary anterior teeth.

(a) Which disease has produced this complaint and this appearance?

(b) How could the gingival recession labial to 11 be treated to improve the appearance?

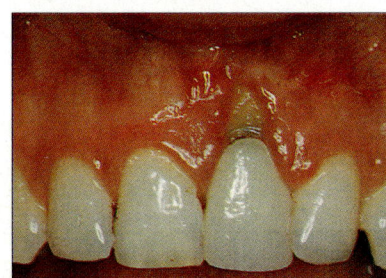

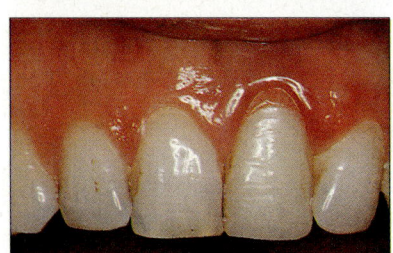

**12** This 25-year-old patient had an apicectomy 1 year ago on 21. Not only has this failed (there is a sinus present between the chronic apical abscess and the gingival margin) but the bone overlying the labial surface of the root was removed during the operative procedure, leaving the patient with unsightly recession. This is apparent when she smiles, causing her embarrassment. She is unwilling to lose the tooth and have it replaced by a denture.

(a) Why may the apicectomy have failed?

(b) How could her problem be overcome (**12C**)?

**13** (a) What condition is shown here?
(b) What residual problems remain?
(c) What is the incidence of this condition?

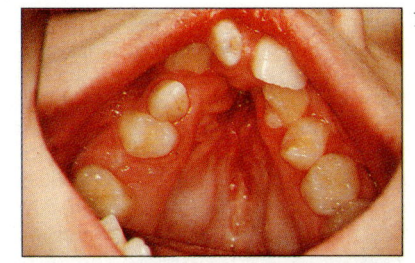

**14** Enumerate the complications of external beam radiotherapy in the treatment of oral malignancy. How should the periodontal tissues be managed before and after radiotherapy ?

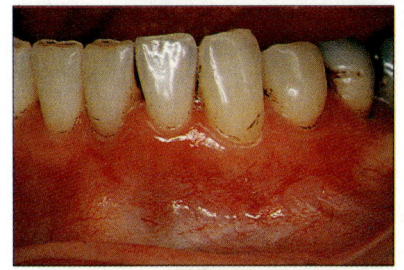

**15** This patient, a 35-year-old female, has periodontitis affecting the upper anterior teeth. Her oral hygiene is now good and the teeth have been root planed twice. Residual pocketing is present and there is still bleeding on probing. You decide that flap surgery is indicated but the patient is anxious that gingival recession is kept to a minimum. How may this be achieved?

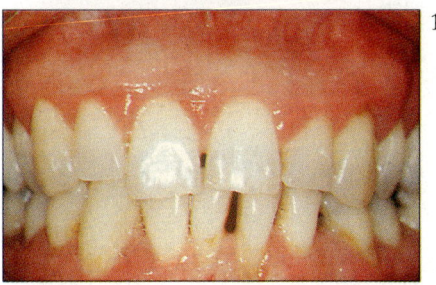

**16** What preventive advice should be given to a patient about to embark on a course of fixed appliance orthodontic treatment?

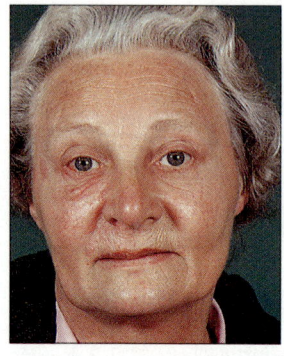

**17** The picture shows an adult patient with a painful vesicular rash along the distribution of a sensory nerve.
(a) What is the name of this condition?
(b) What is the causative agent?
(c) How may the clinical diagnosis be confirmed in the laboratory?
(d) Are there any groups of patients for whom this infection may be particularly dangerous?
(e) Is there any specific treatment available for serious cases?

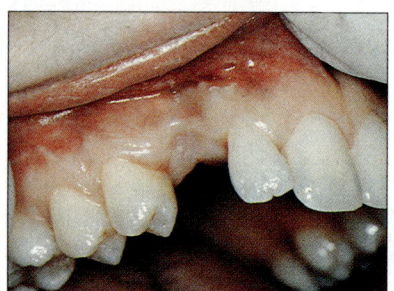

**18** This 23-year-old female had the 13 extracted 1 month previously due to external root resorption. She requests an implant, but there is insufficient bone to support it. How may this be rectified and describe the procedure involved prior to implant placement?

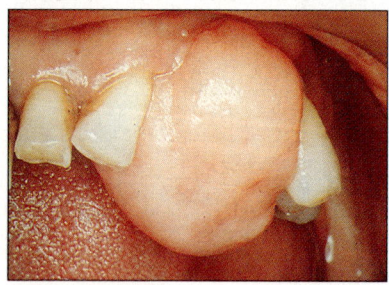

**19** A 52-year-old male, with no relevant medical history or pharmacotherapy, presented with this lesion. The gingival enlargement had been slow-growing over a period of 2 years and, other than that it interfered with his occlusion, was symptomless. The lesion was firm but not hard. Name one simple investigation to assist your diagnosis and the reason for the request. Given that this investigation gave no positive information, what is the most likely diagnosis? Explain why possible alternative diagnoses are less likely to be correct. What was the treatment?

**20** This patient presented with a labial sinus 3mm from the gingival margin of 22 with a history of a repeatedly uncemented post-retained crown in this tooth. A radiograph suggests a root perforation distally. The patient possesses a short post-retained crown.
(a) Describe how this provisional diagnosis would be confirmed.
(b) Describe the treatment of the perforation.

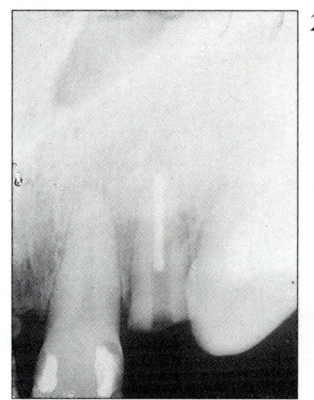

20

**21** This 44-year-old female patient attended the dentist only when she had pain. When this photograph was taken, she had not seen a dentist for several years and the problem of which she was complaining was related to a cariously exposed lower molar. However, the dentist whom she consulted was rightly more concerned about the lesion seen here palatal to the 16. What could the lesion be and what action should be taken concerning it? She admitted to smoking 20 or more cigarettes per day.

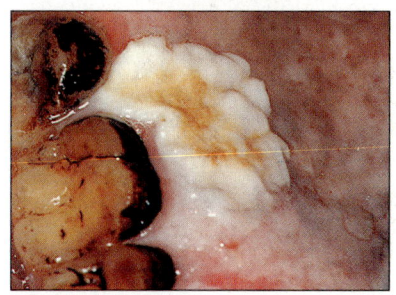

21

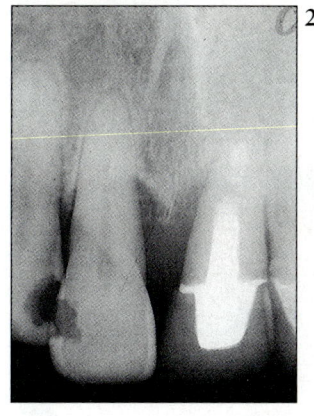

22

**22** (a) What is the term applied to the pattern of bone loss shown here?
(b) How does this pattern of bone loss arise?
(c) How can it be treated?

**23**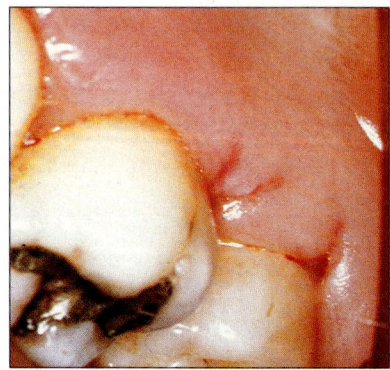

**23** What lesions do you see here and what has caused them?

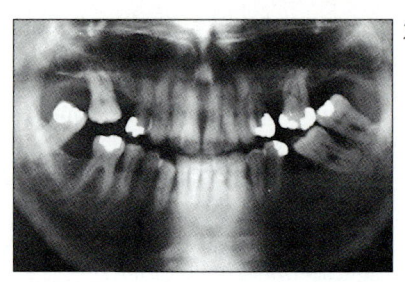
**24**

**24** The orthopantogram of a 38-year-old male presenting with bleeding gums and foetor oris is shown. Indicate your diagnosis and outline the clinical findings you would expect to encounter.

**25**

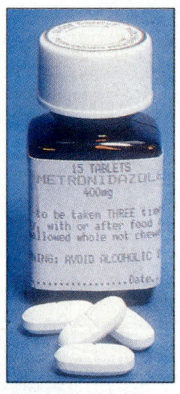

**25** Metronidazole is widely used in the management of adult periodontitis. What are its advantages and unwanted effects?

**26**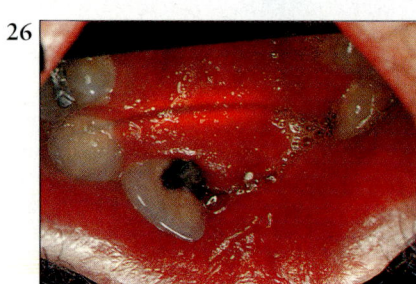

**26** This patient, aged 21, has a repaired cleft of the hard palate. He has worn a succession of removable orthodontic appliances and partial dentures since infancy. He now needs a partial denture in cobalt chromium to replace 21 and 22. The existing partial denture is made of acrylic resin and has full palatal and gingival coverage from 17 to 27. There has been considerable hyperplasia of the palatal gingival tissue but the buccal and labial gum remain unaffected. How may his condition be managed?

**27** A patient presents with a cemented anterior bridge with a symptom-free, non-vital lateral incisor abutment. The radiograph is shown. What is the diagnosis?

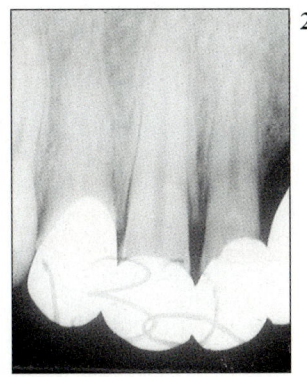

**28** (a) Name this commonly used periodontal dressing.
(b) What are its constituents?
(c) Why are such dressings used?
(d) What are the ideal properties of a periodontal dressing?
(e) Give examples of other types of periodontal packs.

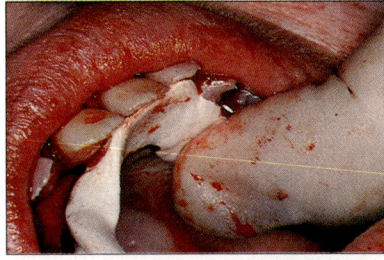

**29** This patient, a 35-year-old male, complained of persistent gingival bleeding from the papilla between 45 and 46. This was not excessive in terms of the quantity of blood, being perhaps more accurately described as oozing. Nevertheless it had persisted for 48 hours. On questioning the patient revealed that he had felt unwell for the previous 2 weeks and had been lethargic and unable to pursue his sporting activities (he was a football referee). The only other oral abnormality was the ecchymosis seen between 21 and 22. What is the likely diagnosis and how should the patient be managed?

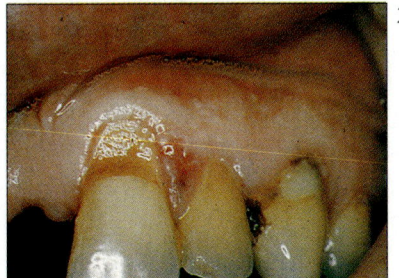

**30**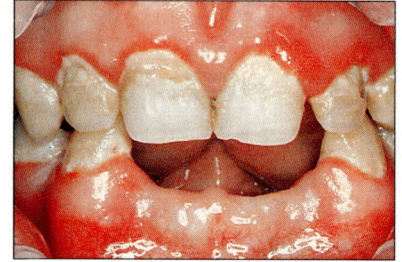

**30** This patient is suffering from plaque-induced gingival inflammation (in addition to a number of other problems).
(a) Give 4 factors in dental plaque that are known to produce gingival damage.
(b) From where do the lipopolysaccharides in plaque arise?
(c) What damage do they cause to the gingival tissues?
(d) What laboratory methods have been shown to be effective in removing lipopolysaccharides?

**31**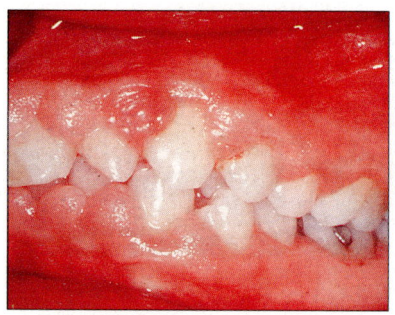

**31** This 60-year-old female patient has gingival enlargement which has been increasing in size over the past 2 years. She has a medical history of angina. What is the likely cause of the gingival enlargement and how would you manage the case?

**32**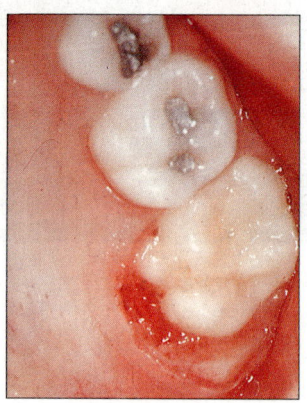

**32** The mother of this 6-year-old child was concerned about this area close to the newly erupting first permanent molar.
(a) What has produced this appearance and what term is usually applied to it?
(b) How would you manage the patient?

**33** Following the sudden onset of fever and a sore throat lasting 2 days, a young child develops multiple, small papulovesicular lesions on the anterior fauces, uvula and soft palate. This condition continues for about 3 or 4 days, after which the fever drops and the oral lesions start to heal. No comparable lesions can be seen on the skin. Several other children at the same nursery school are similarly affected.

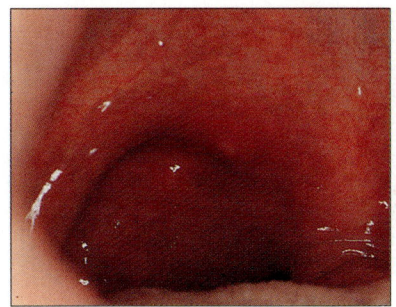

(a) What is the name of this condition?
(b) What is the causative agent?
(c) What rare oral complication may occur and be confused with another childhood viral infection?
(d) What laboratory investigations will confirm the diagnosis?

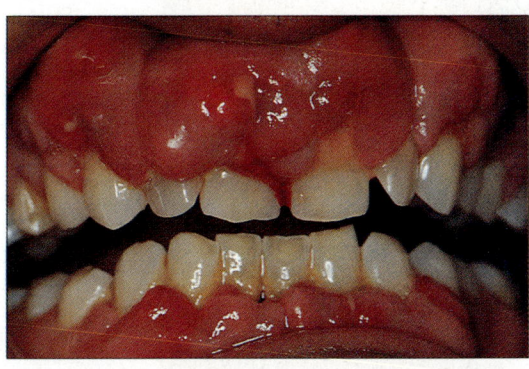

**34** This 56-year-old patient who was not a regular dental attender is complaining of severe pain affecting all his teeth and jaws. This has been present for 2 days. His gums are grossly enlarged and tender to the touch, with pus exuding from some gingival margins. Many areas of the gum—notably that in the upper incisor region—are fluctuant. The teeth and gingival tissues are all very tender to the touch. Gross deposits of sub- and supragingival calculus can be detected. His temperature is elevated and submandibular and submental lymph nodes are enlarged and tender. What is the condition and how may the patient be managed?

**35**

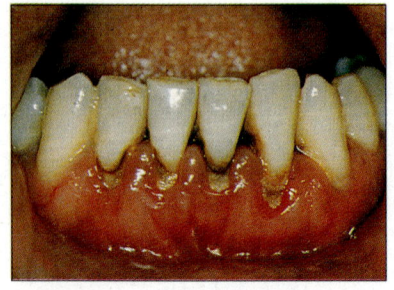

35 (a) What types of calculus can be seen on the labial surfaces of the lower incisor teeth? What criteria do you use to recognise these?
(b) What score would you give to the lower left central incisor (31) using the Calculus Score or the Oral Hygiene Index (Greene and Vermillion, 1960)?
(c) How does the Retention Index (Biorby and Loe, 1967) differ from the Calculus Score?

**36**

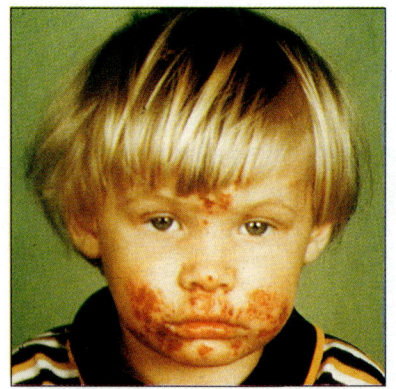

36 This 3-year-old boy has suffered from eczema since birth. This is treated by betamethasone cream. Two days ago he became ill, feverish and extremely lethargic, with a very sore mouth. His eczema became much worse and crusting has started to develop. His mother has been applying the betamethasone cream to his face with increased frequency. How would you establish a diagnosis and how should he be treated?

**37**

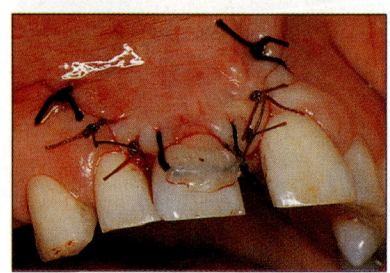

37 (a) The previously exposed root surface of the labial aspect of 11 has been covered by what surgical technique?
(b) What other mucogingival surgical procedure may have been performed prior to this operation, and why?
(c) What additional measures have been used during this type of procedure in order to create a new connective tissue attachment to the exposed root surface?

**38** What are the direct and predisposing aetiological factors demonstrated here?

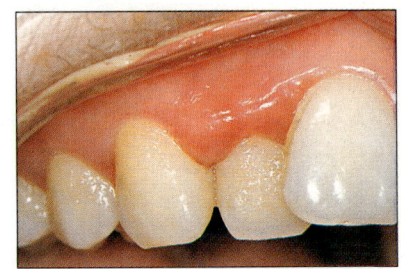

**39** This is a scanning electron micrograph of the buccal cervical region of a tooth exhibiting dentine hypersensitivity. How is the appearance relevant to the considered mechanism for stimulus transmission across dentine? How important is the size of the holes to that mechanism? List ways in which a desensitising toothpaste might stop dentine hypersensitivity.

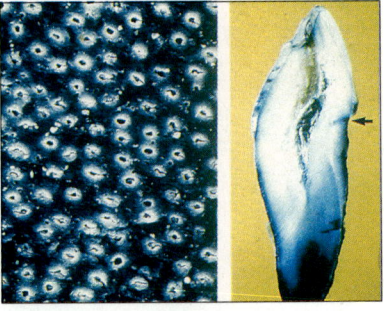

**40** What are the active ingredients of this commercial mouthrinse and how do they exert their action?

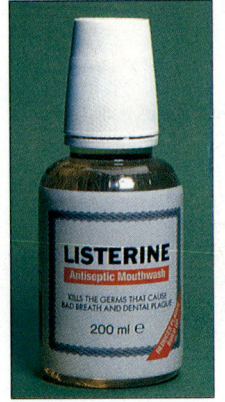

**41** Your trainee DSA receives a needlestick injury when she is re-sheathing the needle after administration of a local anaesthetic. What action should you take? What steps should be taken to avoid a recurrence?

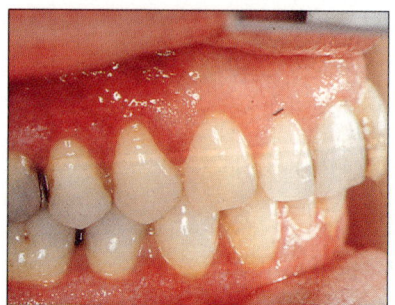

42A

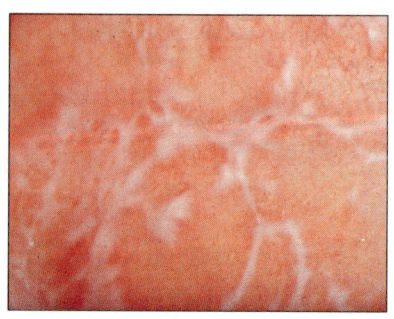

42B

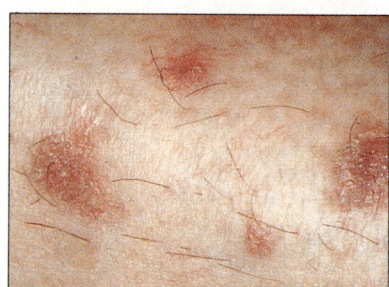

42C

**42** This 45-year-old female presented with 'desquamative gingivitis' and these lesions on her shins (**42C**).
(a) What is the likely underlying cause of her desquamative gingivitis?
(b) What is the underlying histology?

43

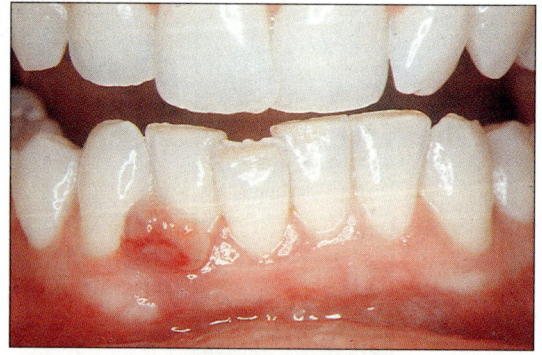

**43** This patient, who is 5 months pregnant, had the epulis associated with the 43 removed 1 month previously. It has now recurred. This is not uncommon when such lesions are surgically removed during pregnancy.
(a) What steps would you take to ensure as far as possible that such a lesion does not recur when removed during pregnancy?
(b) What are the salient histological features of a pregnancy epulis?

**44** This patient and her parents are very concerned about her 'gummy' appearance.
(a) What factors contribute to this?
(b) What treatment would you advise?

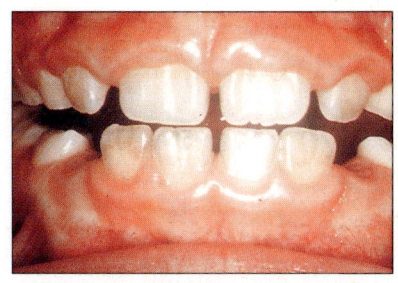

**45** This photograph shows an anti-microbial agent being delivered into a periodontal pocket in a slow release vehicle. What other local method may be used to deliver antimicrobials into periodontal pockets? What are the potential advantages of local compared to systemic delivery of antimicrobials? What potential disadvantages are shared by local and systemic delivery of antimicrobials?

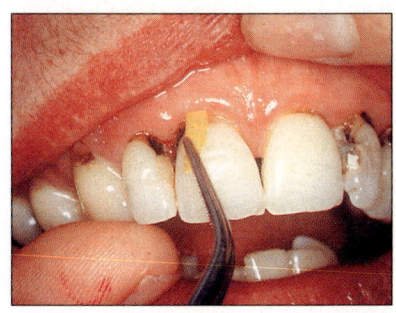

**46** This 17-year-old female patient was concerned about the sensitive upper central incisor teeth and the painful gum between the incisors. Examination of the palatal surfaces of the upper incisor teeth shows evidence of wear of enamel related to the functional contact of the lower incisors. Where dentine had become exposed, it was lost preferentially to the surrounding enamel.
(a) What is the differential diagnosis of the tooth wear?
(b) How should the patient's complaint be addressed?

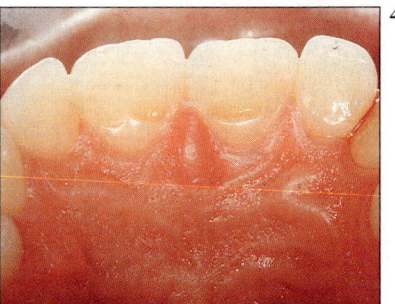

**47**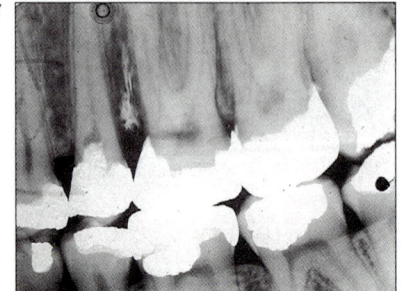

**47** The day before this radiograph was taken, this 22-year-old patient had had a gold inlay cemented in 26. The impression had been taken 2 days before that, using polysulphide rubber. She was complaining of severe pain and the gum overlying the 25, 26 interspace was bright red. How would you account for the appearance of the radiograph?

**48**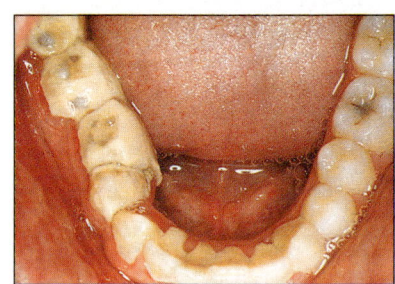

**48** What is the reason for the unusual distribution of calculus in this young male ?

**49A**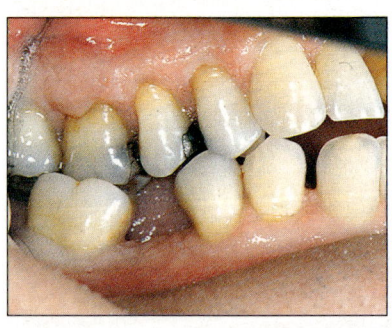

**49B**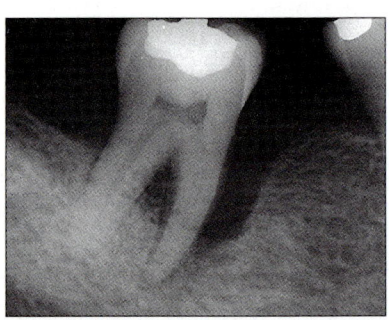

**49** The patient seen in **49A** lost 46 some years ago and wonders whether the gap can be bridged. His radiograph is seen in **49B**. What can be done to help him? 47 reacts positively to vitality testing.

**50** On clinical examination a 45-year-old man showed no periodontal pocketing around 11 but the tooth was Grade 3 mobile. A periapical radiograph was taken.
(a) What features are visible radiographically?
(b) What is the diagnosis?
(c) How may this condition be treated if the patient insists on retaining the tooth?

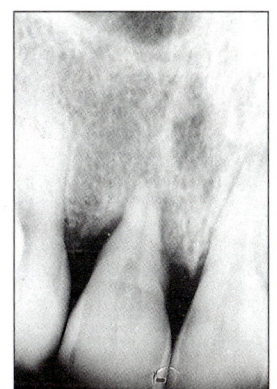

**50**

**51** The mother of this 3-year-old boy brought him to the surgery complaining of spontaneous bleeding from his gums. He had also had several nosebleeds and had recently become very lethargic. On examination his skin and mucosa were very pale. A routine haematological screening was carried out and a diagnosis of leukaemia was made.

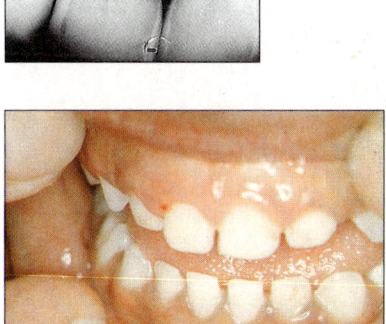

**51**

(a) What type of leukaemia is this likely to be and what would the general features of the haematology report show?
(b) What systemic treatment will he require?
(c) How would you manage his oral care?

**52** The greyish lesion between 35 and 34 has been present for 5 years. The tissues are soft to the touch and not swollen. The lesion appears stable in both consistency and size. It first appeared after the restoration of 35.
(a) What is this lesion?
(b) How does this type arise?
(c) What special test should you do?
(d) What treatment should you give?

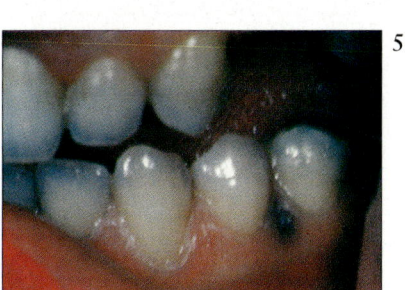

**52**

**53**

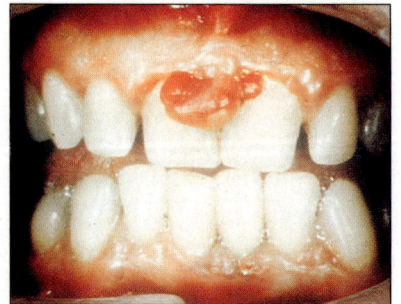

**53** A 22-year-old female who is 6 months pregnant presents with this localised gingival enlargement. The lesion bleeds on minimal trauma as do several other gingival sites. What is the commonly used term to describe this gingival enlargement and the generalised gingival problem? What is the aetiology of the lesion? Suggest possible approaches to management.

**54**

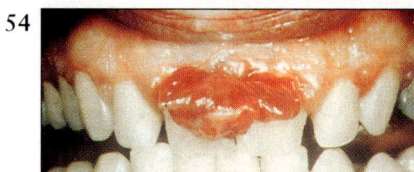

**54** This is the same patient as in **53**, but seen 2 weeks later. Give the reasons in favour of removing pregnancy epulides during pregnancy.

**55**

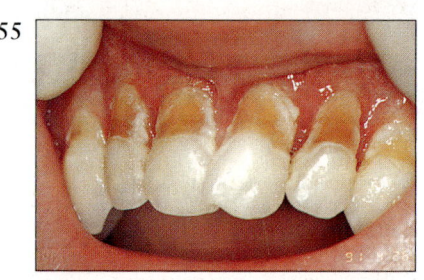

**55** This 4-year-old child has generalised bleeding gums, mobile teeth and no history of trauma. What is your likely diagnosis and what other clinical findings would you expect?

**56**

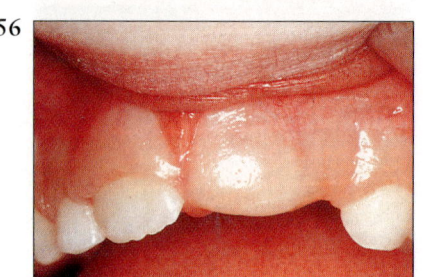

**56** (a) What is the swelling overlying the left upper permanent central incisor known as?
(b) What is the histological appearance?
(c) What treatment is required?

**57** This illustration shows an air polisher being used, producing a copious aerosol. What are the advantages and disadvantages of these instruments and how is the problem of aerosol production best overcome?

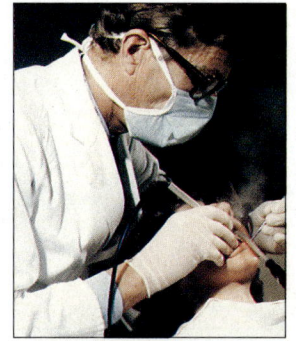

57

**58** What are these instruments and what are they used for?

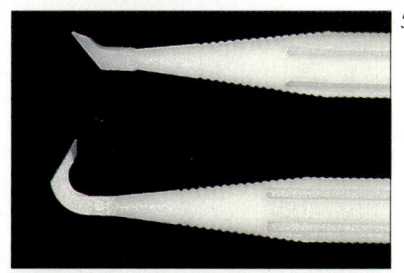

58

**59** What type of probe is this and what are its special features?

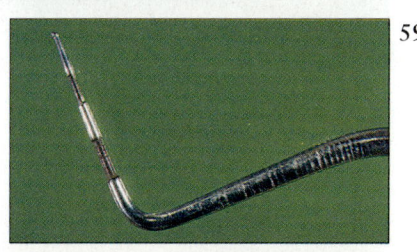

59

**60** This patient's upper first molar has had the disto-buccal root resected. What are the indications for root resection in an upper molar?

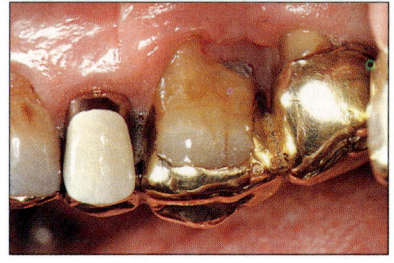

60

**61**

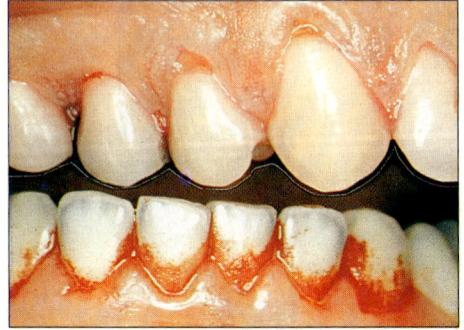

**61** The two subjects shown in this composite photograph are taking part in a plaque growth project. Both had their teeth thoroughly polished to remove all plaque 24 hours before the photographs were taken. Allowing for the fact that the subject in the upper part of the photograph has been disclosed with erythrosin and the one in the lower part with neutral red, which stains more deeply, it is clear that the subject in the lower part of the photograph has grown more plaque than the other. What is the reason for this and is it of any clinical significance?

**62**

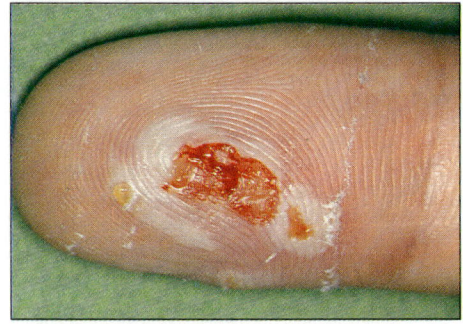

**62** This lesion on the finger of a dentist has been present for 5 days. It is very painful and becoming worse. What is the diagnosis? What precautions should be taken to avoid such infection?

**63** This dried specimen shows two abnormalities of alveolar bone. What are they and what is their significance in relation to periodontal disease?

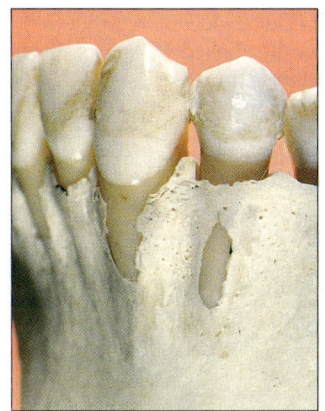

63

**64** Osseointegrated implants *in situ* after removal of the fixed superstructure.
(a) What does the term osseointegration imply?
(b) Between what materials and bone has osseointegration been shown to occur?
(c) What instruments would be used to remove the deposits of calculus shown in the picture?
(d) What steps could the patient take to prevent the calculus reforming after it had been removed?

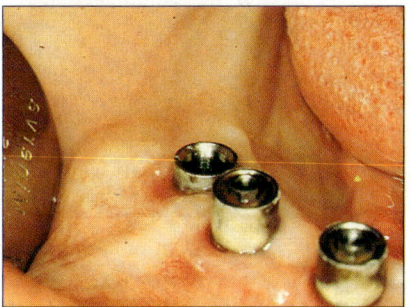

64

**65** What are the features of post-operative pain after periodontal surgery? How is such pain best managed?

**66** Chlorhexidine gluconate, either in the form of a 0·2% mouthrinse solution or as a topically applied 1% gel, is sometimes used as an antiseptic for various oral conditions.
(a) What is the spectrum of activity of this antimicrobial agent against oral micro-organisms?
(b) Is any clinically significant species of oral bacteria known to be particularly sensitive to chlorhexidine?
(c) What is the mode of action of chlorhexidine against bacteria?
(d) Are there any other factors which appear to enhance the efficacy of chlorhexidine as an oral antiseptic?
(e) What are the possible disadvantages or side-effects of long-term use of chlorhexidine in the mouth?

**67**

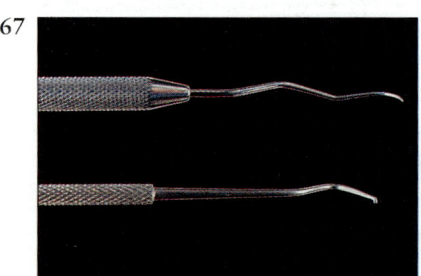

**67** What are these instruments used for?

**68**

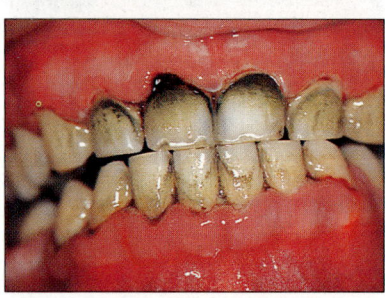

**68** What may account for the unusual green stain on the teeth of this 47-year-old patient? He has not had them professionally cleaned for some years but claims to brush his teeth daily.

**69** This 6-year-old boy was complaining of bleeding from the gums around his newly erupting incisor teeth.
(a) What investigations would you carry out?
(b) What treatment would you advise?
(c) Give a differential diagnosis.

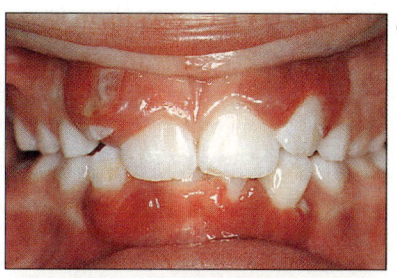

**70** What is this brush used for? What other methods are available for this purpose?

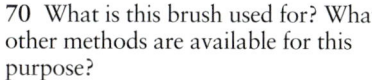

**71** What is the explanation for the unusual appearance of this patient's teeth?

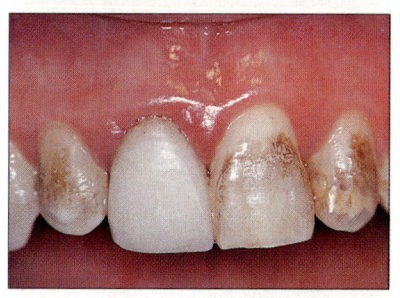

**72** The lower right first molar in this 40-year-old black woman has a periodontal/endodontic lesion involving the distal apex. What is the differential diagnosis of the radio-opaque lesion associated with the mesial apex?

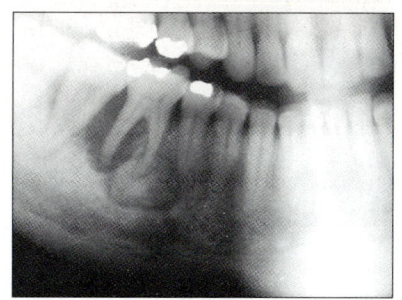

**73**

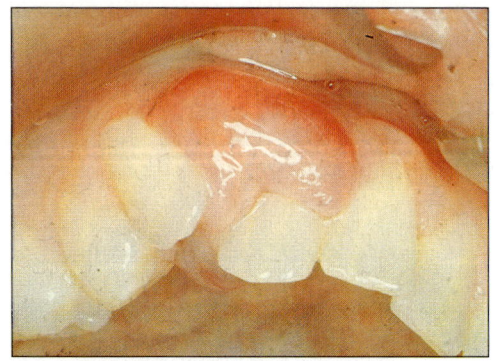

**73** This 27-year-old female presented with the swelling shown. She was 8 months pregnant and described the lesion as having been present for approximately 6 months. At first it had apparently increased in size but for the 4 weeks prior to presentation it had not changed. The lesion was otherwise symptomless. Given only this clinical information and appearance, suggest possible diagnoses and how you would manage the condition. Would you modify or firm up your diagnosis if post-partum the lesion did not spontaneously reduce in size? What two investigations would you request post-partum and what might these reveal?

**74**

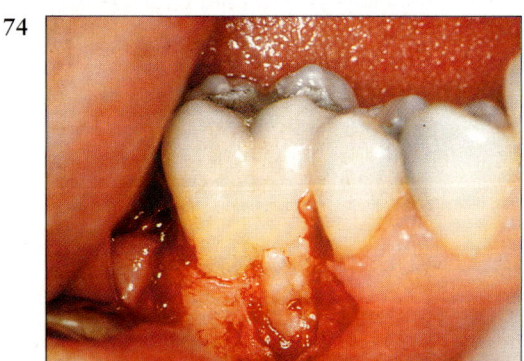

**74** This patient gave a history of recurrent acute abscesses on the buccal side of 46. On examination a pocket was found with a hard protuberance on the root surface. It was decided to raise a flap to explore the area. What is the abnormality and how would you proceed?

**75** What are the problems of prescribing drugs to a breast-feeding mother? What drugs used in dentistry should be avoided in such patients?

**76** This patient has been suffering from severe refractory periodontitis, and 12 months previously had been provided with a fixed Rochette-type splint to control excess mobility.

(a) What would be the diagnosis, given the information on the radiograph?

(b) What further investigations should be undertaken?

(c) What treatment could be provided to save this tooth?

(d) What types of restoration would be possible if this tooth were lost?

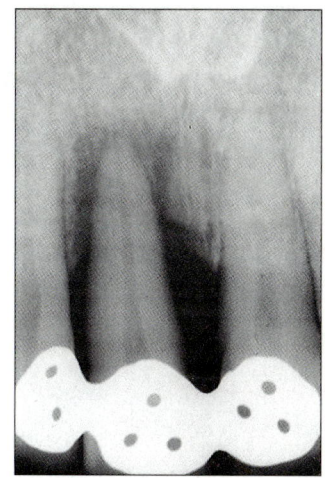

**77** This lesion of the buccal mucosa presented in a 28-year-old male. It was symptomless and had been present as long as he could remember. The surface was soft and when removed it left normal epithelium below.

(a) What is the diagnosis and histology?

(b) How should this condition be treated?

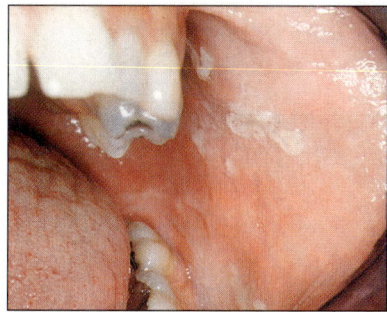

**78** What feature is shown on this radiograph that will affect the prognosis of the first molar?

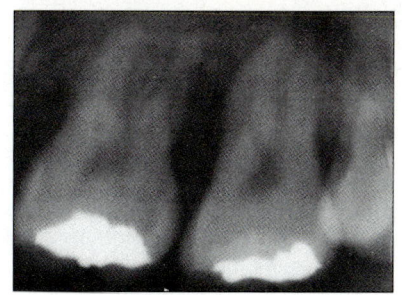

**79**

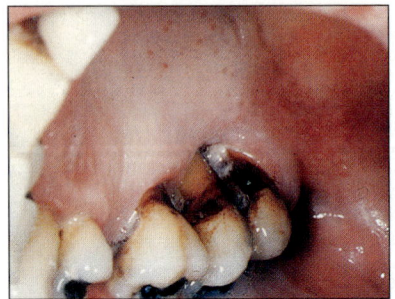

79 This patient, who is HIV-positive, has a related periodontal condition. Diagnose the condition. List the clinical features.

**80**

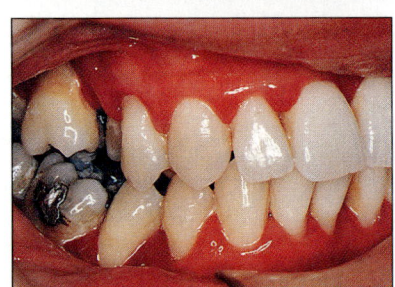

80 This 17-year-old girl complained of gingival soreness, oral ulceration and upper respiratory tract infections occurring at 3-weekly intervals.
(a) What is the most likely diagnosis?
(b) What laboratory investigations would you carry out to establish the diagnosis?
(c) How would you treat her?

**81A**

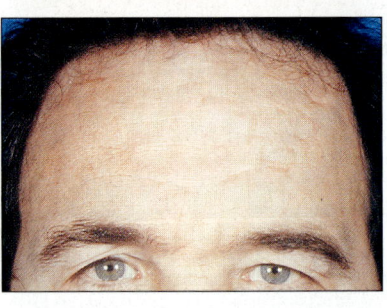

**81B**

81 This patient presented with a loose lower incisor tooth. Radiographs show unusually shaped pulp chambers and clinical examination demonstrated multiple scarring of the skin in exposed areas and hypermobility of the joints.
(a) What is the syndrome?
(b) What is the form of inheritance most frequently encountered in this rare condition?
(c) What dental problems are there?

**82** This 40-year-old male patient has pocketing of over 6mm at many sites including the upper anterior region shown. Assuming that the preventive phase of management has been achieved thus far and the patient is practising a high standard of oral hygiene, what is the primary aim of the treatment phase? What would be the reason for non-surgical (root planing) as opposed to surgical treatment methods and vice versa?

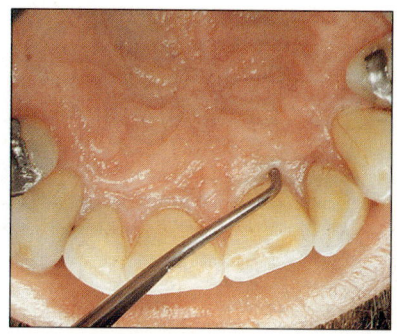

**83** (a) What procedures have been undertaken in the patient shown?
(b) What advice would you give this patient concerning the care of the mouth?
(c) What advice should you give concerning the removable prosthesis?
(d) What are the advantages of this type of prosthesis over a conventional one?

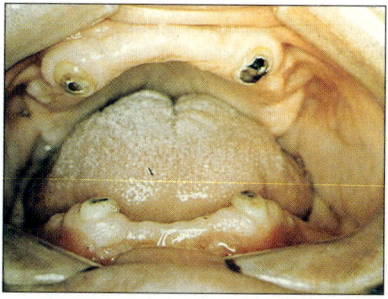

**84** 'Periodontal disease is a slowly progressive, chronic inflammatory disease process, starting at the gum margin and spreading if unchecked to involve the alveolar bone and periodontal ligament resulting in eventual loss of teeth.'

This was once regarded as a satisfactory definition of plaque-induced periodontal disease. Modern knowledge suggests that it is now outmoded. What are the present day concepts of periodontal disease and its progression?

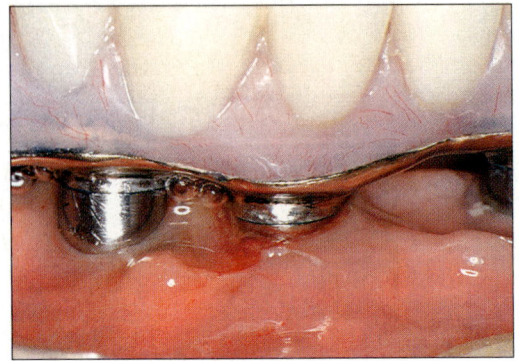

**85** An edentulous 50-year-old woman who has had a lower implant-retained bridge for over 2 years attends with 'toothache' and swollen gum around the implant in the area of a few days duration.
(a) How would you investigate the condition?
(b) What is the most likely diagnosis?
(c) What aetiological and predisposing factors may be involved?
(d) How should the condition be treated?

86

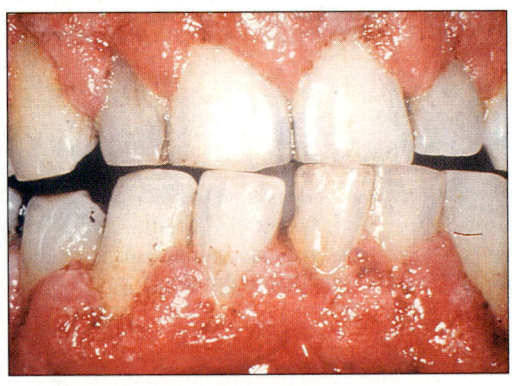

**86** A 64-year-old male presented for investigation and treatment of this unusual gingival hyperplasia. What investigations would you carry out?

**87** What effect does smoking have on the periodontal tissues and their response to plaque?

**88** (a) What mechanisms of loss of tooth substance may have been involved here?
(b) How will you investigate the patient's complaint of excessive tooth wear?

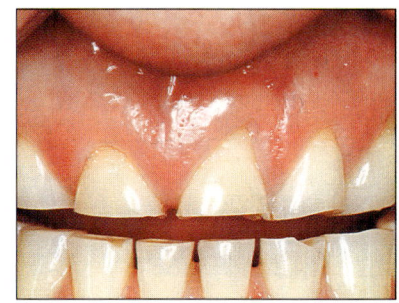

**89** This unusual appearance of the palate was noticed in a 36-year-old male patient who had a history of asthma.
(a) What is the diagnosis ?
(b) How may this have arisen ?
(c) What advice/treatment should be administered ?
(d) If this clinical condition were resistant to conventional therapy, what underlying condition should be suspected ?

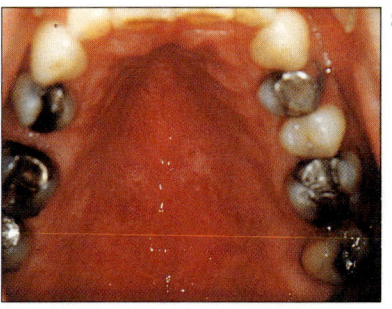

**90** What is the significance of this girl's malocclusion to her periodontal health?

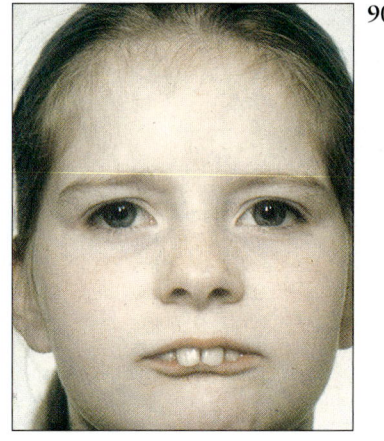

**91** You are administering a local anaesthetic and the patient complains of feeling light-headed and unwell. What is the possible cause and how should the patient be managed?

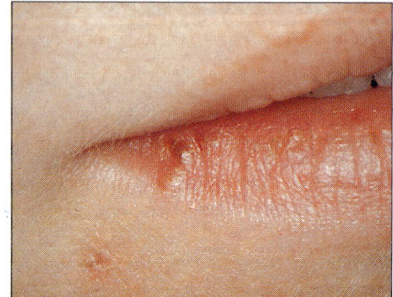

**92** What is this lesion on the lip of a dentist? What precautions should she take when treating patients and is any treatment possible for it?

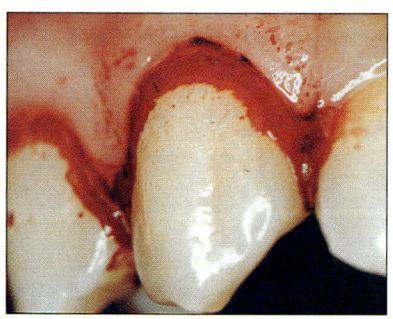

**93** What would the plaque score be for this canine using:
(a) The plaque index (Silness and Löe, 1964);
(b) Modified Plaque Index (Walsh *et al.*, 1992);
(c) Oral Hygiene Index (Greene and Vermilion, 1960);and
(d) Patient Hygiene Performance (Podshadley and Haley, 1968).

**94** Two types of periodontal lesion have been described in association with human immunodeficiency virus (HIV) infection, a generalised atypical gingivitis (HIV-gingivitis; HIV-G) and a rapidly progressive periodontitis (HIV-periodontitis; HIV-P).
(a) Does HIV-G respond as readily as gingivitis in HIV-negative patients to conventional dental plaque removal and improved oral hygiene procedures?
(b) Is the microbial flora associated with HIV-G any different to that found in HIV-negative subjects with gingivitis?
(c) Is there any evidence that HIV-G lesions are precursors of the tissue destruction observed in HIV-P?
(d) Are there any similarities between HIV-P and ANUG in HIV negative subjects?
(e) Which periodontopathic bacteria have been detected in subgingival plaque samples from patients with HIV-G and HIV-P?

**95** The picture shows an oral ulcer in a patient with chicken pox.
(a) What is the causative agent of chicken pox?
(b) What other clinical manifestations of chicken pox are normal, particularly in children?
(c) Do any other childhood fevers cause oral changes?
(d) What other clinical condition is produced by the causative agent of chicken pox, particularly in adults?

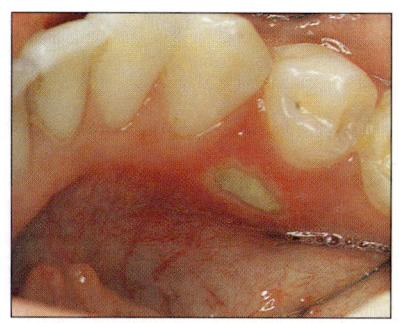
95

**96** Upon examination of this HIV positive patient, a white lesion on the lateral border of the tongue was noted. The lesion was asymptomatic, had not been noticed by the patient and could not be removed by scraping.
(a) State the clinical nomenclature given to the lesion.
(b) What is the proposed viral aetiology?
(c) Why is this lesion important?
(d) What other conditions mimic this clinical presentation?

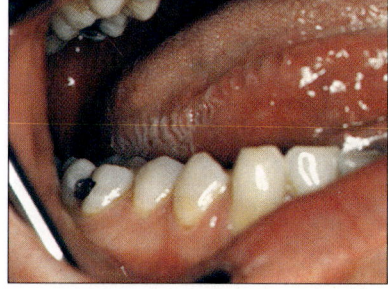
96

**97** This adult female patient presented with a sore mouth and lips of sudden onset. The attached gingiva is bright red and tender. What is your likely diagnosis? What investigations would you carry out and how would you treat this condition?

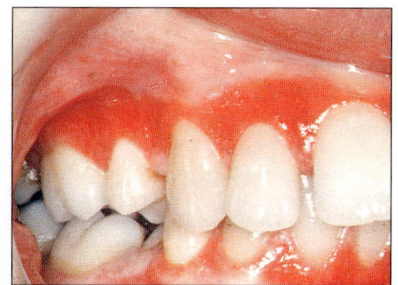
97

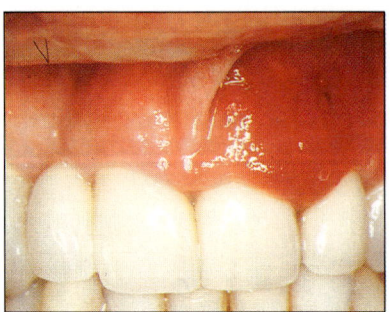 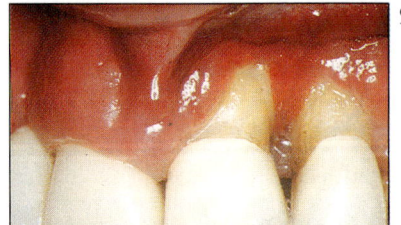

98A 98B

**98** This mildly painful lesion presented in a 38-year-old male with an otherwise clear medical history. The patient had first become aware of it 3 months previously. It was soft and 'velvet-like' to palpate and there was no radiographic evidence of bone involvement.
(a) What is the differential diagnosis ?
(b) How would the diagnosis be confirmed ?
(c) The lesion was in fact (a)(ii) (in Answer section). How should this patient be managed?

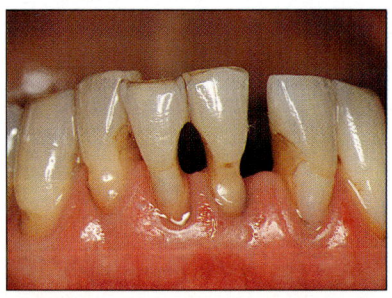

99

**99** What is the explanation for the curious appearance of these lower incisors in a 63-year-old female patient? How can further tooth substance loss be minimised?

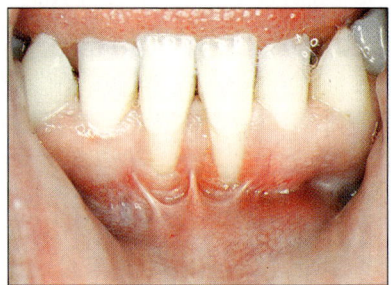

100

**100** (a) What problems may be caused by these mandibular fraenal attachments?
(b) What oral hygiene measures could you recommend?
(c) What treatment may be provided for this condition?
(d) What procedure will reliably give an increase in the depth of the vestibular sulcus in this situation?

**101** The mother of this 3-month-old healthy baby is very concerned about the lumps that she has observed in his mouth.
(a) What are they?
(b) How common are they?
(c) What treatment would you advise?

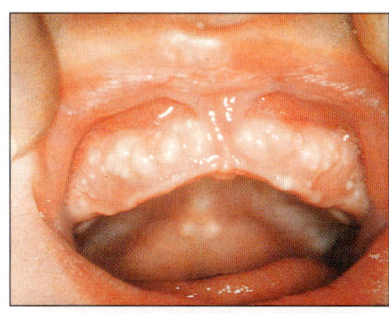

**101**

**102** The instrument on the bottom is a universal curette while that on the top is a Gracey curette. How do the two differ?

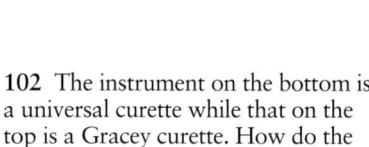

**102**

**103** This 50-year-old female patient is complaining of pain and soreness of her gums, which have been present for about one year. On examination you find that the epithelium can easily be scraped off the underlying tissues. What is the probable diagnosis and how should the patient be managed?

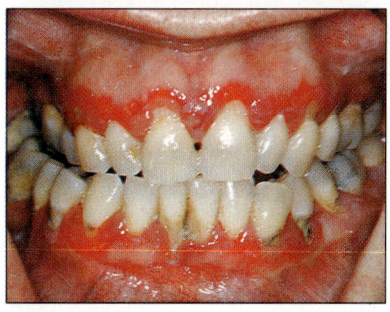

**103**

**104** What are the advantages of using gingival crevicular fluid analysis over conventional methods in the diagnosis of the periodontal diseases?

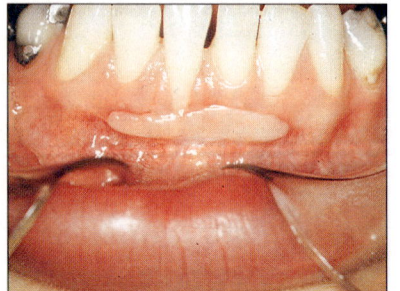

**105** (a) What procedure has been carried out in this patient's lower incisor region to account for the unusual gingival appearance?
(b) What are the stages involved in this technique?

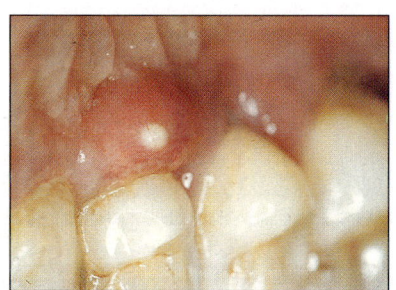

**106** (a) What are the two most likely causes of the sinus shown here?
(b) What special tests would help in making a definitive diagnosis?
(c) Assuming this is a periodontal problem, give five possible reasons why suppuration occurs in this situation.
(d) What periodontal treatment could you provide for this tooth?

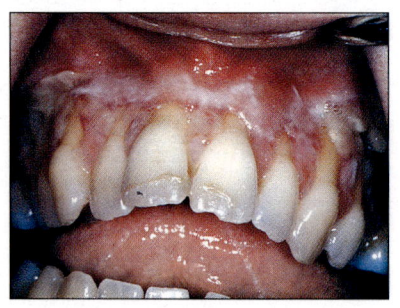

**107** A 32-year-old female under medical treatment for psychiatric illness presents in your surgery complaining of sensitivity in her teeth, gingival recession and sore gums.
(a) What is the most likely diagnosis?
(b) How would you treat this case?

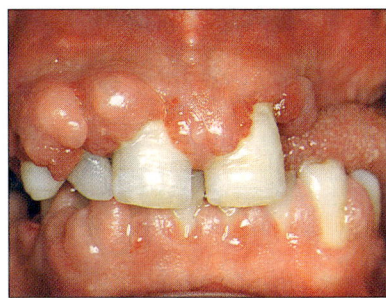 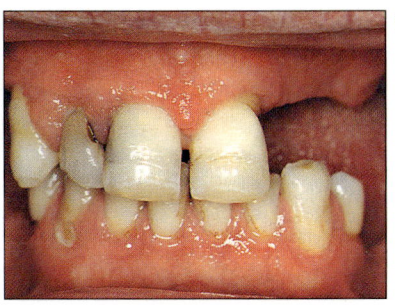

**108** Two years ago this patient underwent heart transplantation. His drug therapy included cyclosporin and nifedipine. His complaint was that the gingival enlargement was unsightly and that he could no longer wear his upper partial denture. **108B** shows him one year later. How might this result have been achieved?

**109** This patient attended his dentist 24 hours before this photograph was taken, with toothache. The source of trouble was traced to 25 which was temporarily dressed under local analgesia. What is the likely cause of the lesion affecting the soft tissues in this area?

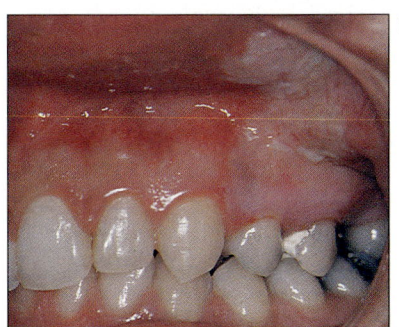

109

**110** (a) What has caused this appearance on the cheek mucosa of this 8-year-old child?
(b) What action is required?

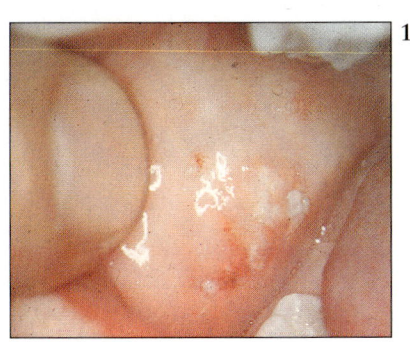

110

**111**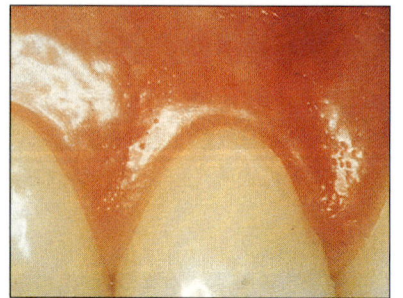

**111** The interdental papilla seen in this picture shows a prominent feature which is said to be a sign of gingival health. What is it and what causes it?

**112**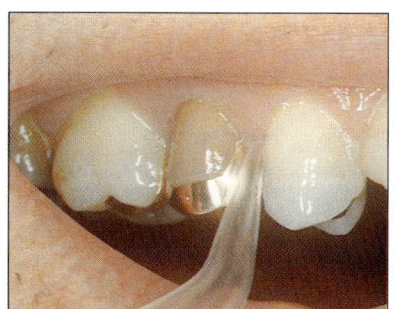

**112** This patient is using a pulsed oral irrigator mesially to this upper second premolar:
(a) Give 4 indications for the use of pulsed oral irrigation.
(b) How does it differ from rinsing as a method of delivering a chemical agent?
(c) What are the hazards of this type of home therapy?
(d) What types of applicator are available for pulsed oral irrigators?

**113**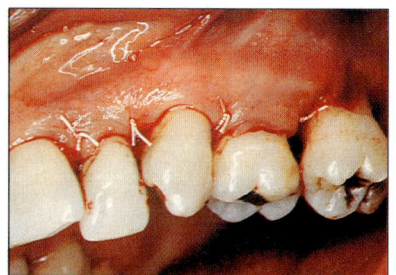

**113** (a) What design of flap procedure has been used in this case?
(b) What are the indications for this type of flap?
(c) What advantages does this technique offer when compared to other periodontal treatment modalities?

**114** This patient underwent renal transplantation some 6 months ago. What is the likely cause of the gingival changes and how would you manage this condition?

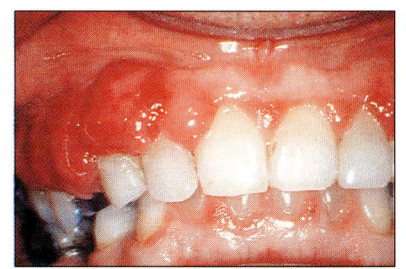

**115** The periodontal condition around this patient's crowned upper incisor is very poor. Indicate why this may be and state what needs to be done before new crowns are constructed. The basic periodontal examination (BPE) score for the sextant is 3.

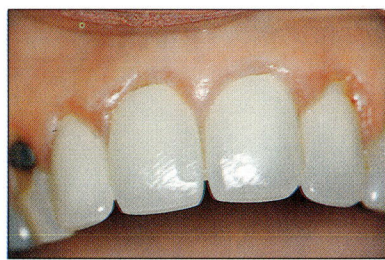

**116** An electrosurgical unit is being used to reduce the gingival tissue distolingual to 47.
(a) Are there any errors evident in the procedure being adopted here?
(b) What particular precautions should be taken when using electrosurgical equipment?

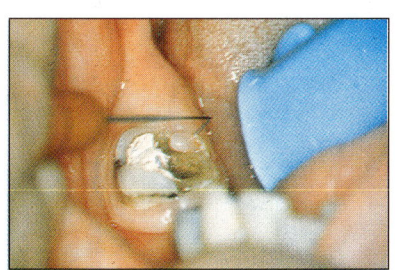

**117** What may be the long-term complications of gingivectomy?

**118**

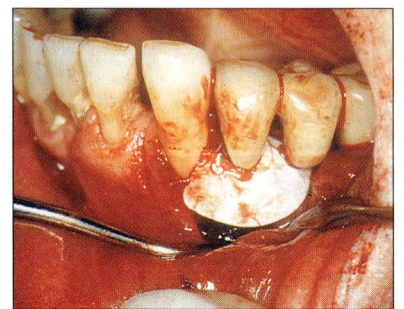

**118** This periodontal/endodontic lesion was treated by guided tissue regeneration (GTR).
(a) What types of membrane are available for this procedure ?
(b) When type 1 (see answer) is used, what is the follow-up period ?
(c) What are the indications for GTR in dentistry ?
(d) What is the main problem with type 2 materials ?

**119**

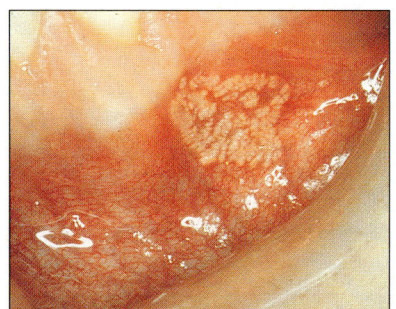

**119** This 25-year-old patient is concerned because he has recently become aware of a symptomless patch in the buccal mucosa. What is:
(a) The diagnosis?
(b) The histology?
(c) The correct treatment?

**120**

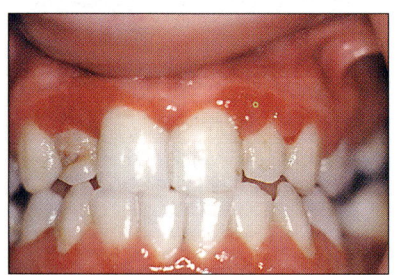

**120** List the clinical changes which would lead you to suspect chronic destructive periodontal disease in this patient. What tests would you instigate to check for loss of periodontal ligament attachment?

**121** This 50-year-old man presented complaining about the appearance of his upper anterior teeth. Apart from some ulceration between the upper incisor teeth, the soft tissues are healthy and the teeth caries-free.
(a) What is your differential diagnosis?
(b) How would you treat him if removal of the etiology was unpredictable?

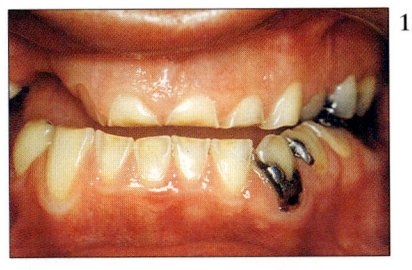
121

**122** This 19-year-old male has no relevant medical history and is not receiving any pharmacotherapy. What is the term given to this common gingival condition? Assuming the condition is mainly localised to the anterior teeth, what local factors could explain this distribution?

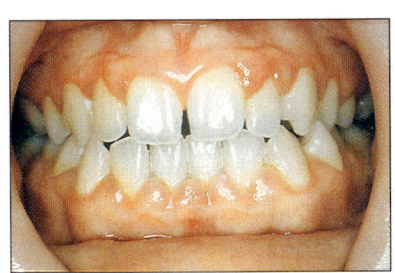
122

**123** This patient is complaining of pain associated with 11. You diagnose an acute abscess. What are the main points of difference between an apical abscess and a lateral periodontal abscess which will help with diagnosis?

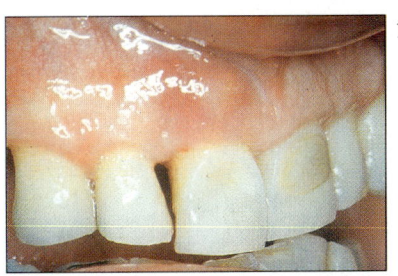
123

**124** A dentist in the United Kingdom who permits a dental hygienist to administer local infiltration analgesia or to work unsupervised must be satisfied that the dental hygienist is competent to do so. In order to be competent to administer local infiltration analgesia what must the dental hygienist have done?

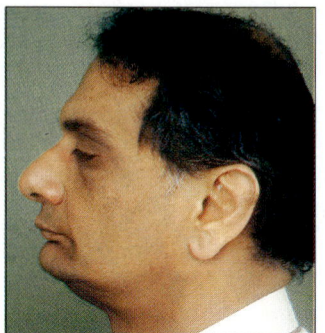 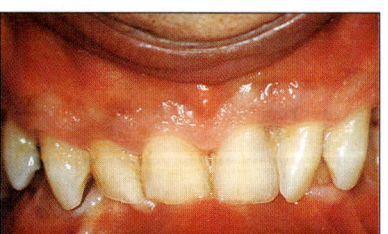

**125** This middle-aged man has a Class II Division II incisal relationship with complete overbite and direct contact with the lower labial gingiva. He presents complaining of tenderness of his lower anterior teeth, painful bleeding gums particularly when awakening and at mealtimes, in addition to a clicking TMJ and occasional limitation of opening. His teeth present are:

<u>17 14 13 12 11  21 22 23 27</u>
  46 44 42 41  31 32 33 34 35 37

  The lower molar and premolar teeth are inclined lingually and all teeth are vital.
(a) Suggest a diagnosis.
(b) What would be an appropriate treatment plan?

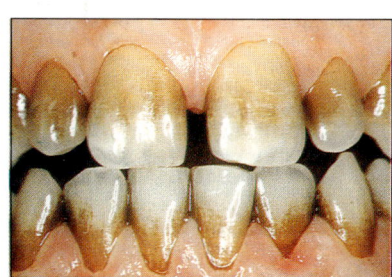

**126** This young man has been rinsing twice a day for 4 weeks with a chlorhexidine mouth rinse. Describe the appearance of the teeth and indicate how this occurs. List the other local side-effects reported with the oral use of chlorhexidine products. Chlorhexidine is used extensively in medicine and dentistry; why then should the antiseptic not be placed into the external auditory meatus?

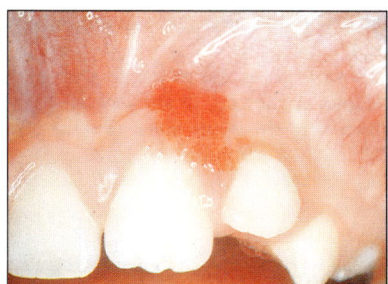
7A

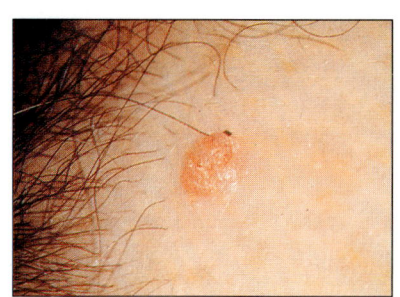
127B

**127** This symptomless lesion was present in a 7-year-old girl. She had been aware of its presence for a month. She had no relevant medical history but gave a history of finger sucking. Radiographs were unremarkable.
(a) What is the differential diagnosis?
(b) How could the diagnosis be established? What relationship is there between the causative agent of this girl's condition and the lesions shown in **127B** and **C**?

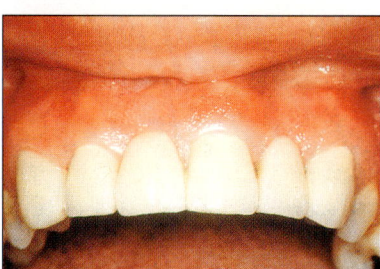
127C

**128** This patient who is HIV-positive has a gingival condition. Indicate the probable diagnosis and describe the clinical features. What treatment would you carry out?

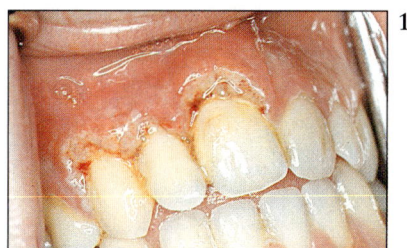
128

**129** What complications may occur during the course of a gingivectomy?

**130**

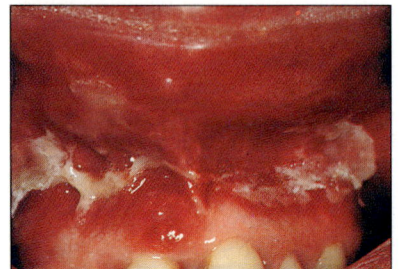

130  This patient is complaining of pain which started 2 days ago, localised to 11. Discomfort has now spread to involve the gingiva and labial mucosa of the upper incisor region. What is the diagnosis and how would you deal with the situation?

**131**

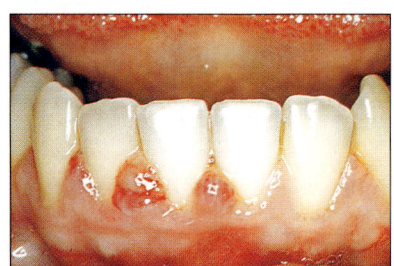

131  This 25-year-old patient is in the fourth month of a normal pregnancy and complains that she has a constant bad taste and that her gums bleed profusely whenever she tries to brush her teeth. What is her condition and how would you manage it?

**132A**

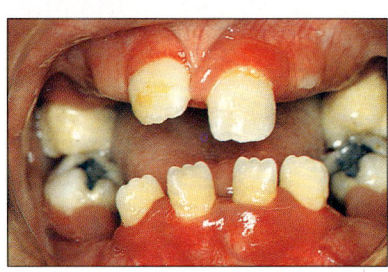

**132B**

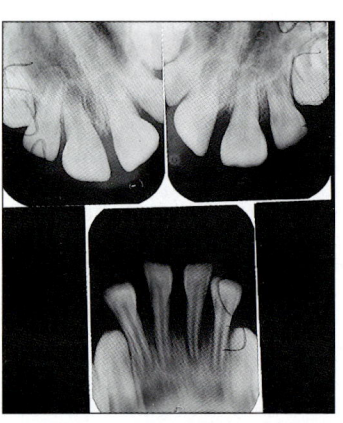

132  All the recently erupted teeth of this 8-year-old boy were very mobile and many primary teeth had exfoliated prematurely. His palmar skin was thickened and fissured.
(a) What is this condition?
(b) How should it be managed?
(c) Suggest differential diagnoses for premature exfoliation of teeth.

**133** (a) What type of probe is this?
(b) What advantages are gained by using this type of probe instead of a standard periodontal probe?

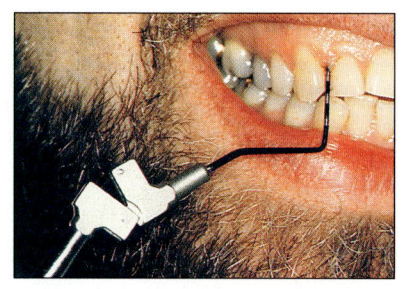

**134** This patient, a 46-year-old man, attended for a routine check. How do you account for the appearance of his palate and how may he be treated?

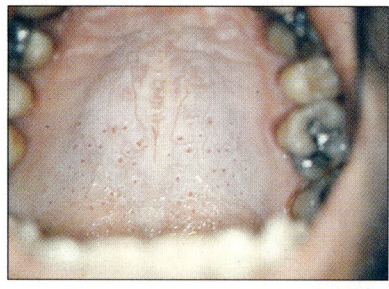

**135** The phenomenon of cavitation is known to occur during ultrasonic scaling:
(a) Give 4 features of cavitation.
(b) Give 5 disadvantages of ultrasonic scaling.
(c) On what types of patients would you avoid using the ultrasonic scaler and why?
(d) What phenomenon other than cavitation occurs in the water around the ultrasonic scaler tip?

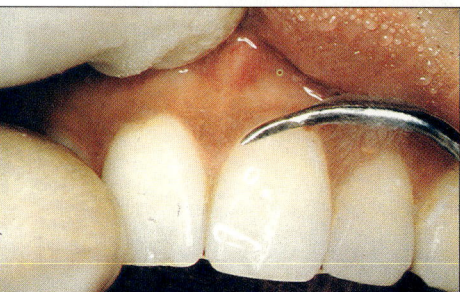

**136**

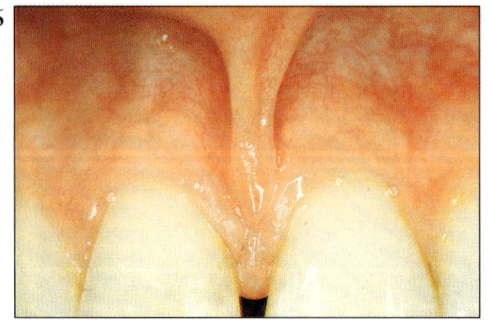

**136** (a) Is the type of maxillary fraenum shown here usually associated with gingival recession?
(b) With what other problems is it known to be associated?
(c) What procedure could be used to remove it? Describe the procedure briefly.

**137A**

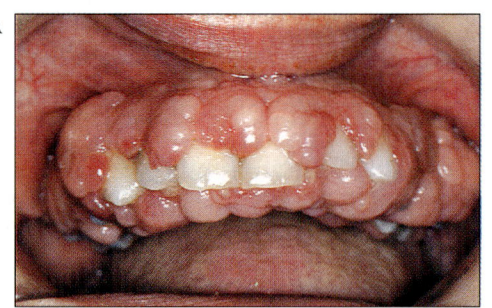

**137B**

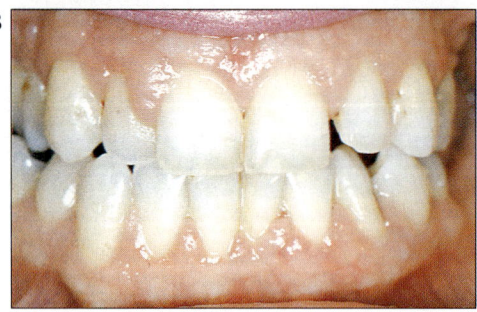

**137** These photographs illustrate the pre-and post-operative gingival appearance of a patient who had had a renal transplant 2 years previously. What is the condition illustrated and what treatment has been administered?

**138** This 19-year-old male presented with painful erosions of the oral mucosa and gingivae and crusting of the lips of sudden onset. There was also ulceration of the penis (**138B**) and red lesions of the palm of the hand (**138C**). He gave a history of a recent bereavement over which he had been under a great deal of stress. His medical practitioner had placed him on anxiolytics and also penicillin for an ear infection. When the oral lesions appeared, he had been placed on prednisolone in an effort to clear up the condition; however this appeared to exacerbate it. Removal of all medication slowly in stages resulted in resolution of the lesions.

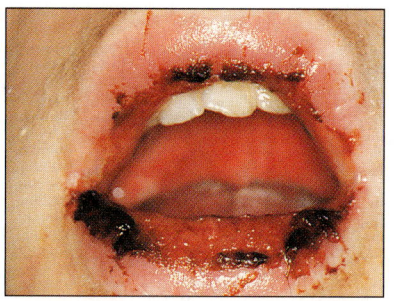
138A

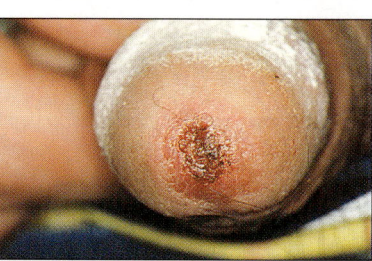
138B

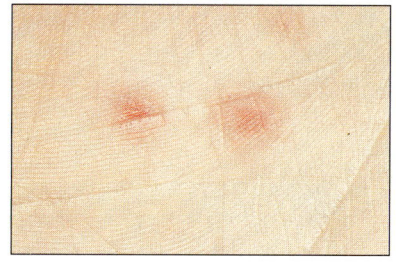
138C

(a) What is this condition and what is the name given to the severe form of this condition ?
(b) What are the reported classical causes of the condition ?
(c) Upon what basis is a diagnosis made ?
(d) In this case what is the likely aetiology ?

**139** A common viral infection can cause acute gingivo-stomatitis in children, with fever, widespread oral ulceration and discomfort, or, alternatively, may produce a mild, sub-clinical infection that is hardly noticeable.
(a) What is the name of this virus?
(b) To what group of viruses does it belong?
(c) What secondary effects are commonly observed after primary infection with this virus?
(d) What laboratory tests may be used to confirm the clinical diagnosis?
(e) Are there any particular hazards or serious consequences associated with this infection?
(f) What specific treatment may be prescribed?

**140**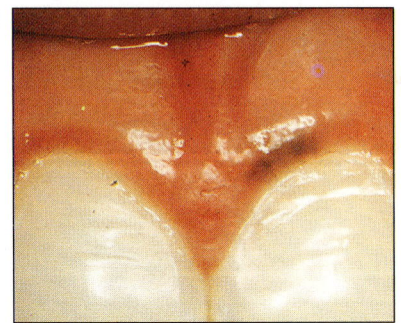

**140** This 19-year-old female student presented with a brown pigmented lesion on the marginal gingivae of the 21, which was of 4 months' duration. The lesion was symptomless and had not enlarged over the previous 3 months. She was a healthy young adult with no history of any medical conditions that are known to give rise to oral pigmentation and there were no other lesions of the oral mucous membranes. What is the differential diagnosis and appropriate management of this case?

**141**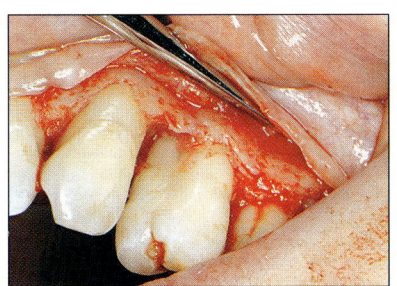

**141** The bone loss on the mesial surface of 24 is more advanced than elsewhere in the mouth. Why might this be? What plaque control procedure would you advise for the patient who is being treated by means of an apically repositioned flap:
(a) In the week following operation?
(b) In the long-term?

**142**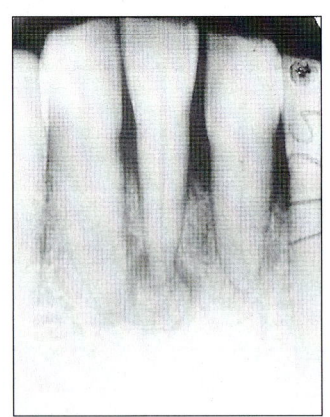

**142** The lesion at the apex of 31 was discovered on routine examination of the lower incisors. All the teeth react positively to vitality testing. What is the likely diagnosis of the lesion and what is the correct treatment?

**143** This 35-year-old male requests the provision of an upper implant to replace the missing 11, 21, 22. An upper acrylic partial denture had been provided 5 years previously following loss of these teeth in a sports injury.

Examination reveals evidence of a high caries rate and denture-associated stomatitis. There are no significant pocket probing depths, but labial recession is evident. The patient is a diet-controlled diabetic but otherwise healthy.

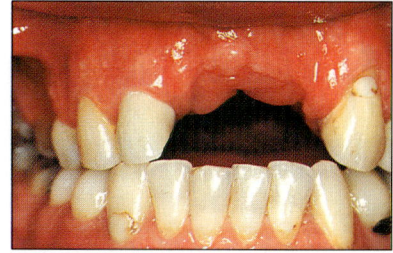

(a) What are the 4 main conditions for the provision of an osseointegrated implant retained bridge for this patient?
(b) What are the medical contraindications to the provision of osseointegrated implants?
(c) What treatment may be provided for the existing problems?
(d) What definitive prosthesis may be provided for this patient?

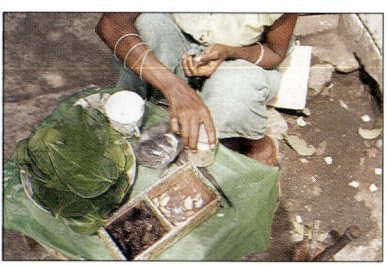

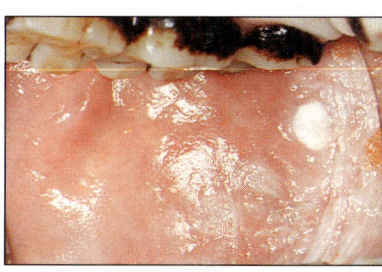

**144** What is the connection between the wares being prepared by the Sri Lankan street trader in **144A** and the lesion shown in **144B**?

**145** (a) How is probing depth defined?
(b) How is pocket depth defined?
(c) How is loss of attachment measured?

**146**

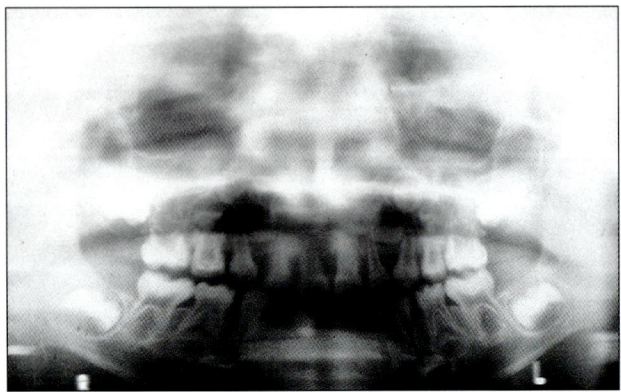

**146** This is the orthopantomograph of an 18-month-old boy, demonstrating premature loss of the deciduous incisor teeth. The teeth exfoliated with complete roots and there was evidence of bone loss to one-third of the root length. There was no other medical history, but at the age of 4 years the child had complained of ankle and foot pains.
(a) What is the likely diagnosis?
(b) How may it be confirmed?
(c) What is the proposed mechanism of tooth loss?
(d) How should the child be managed in future?

**147**

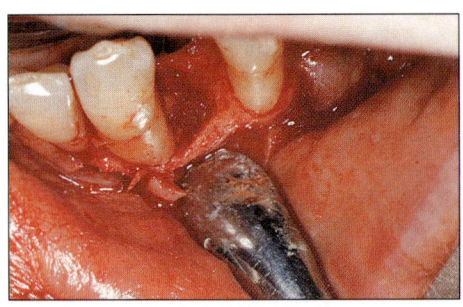

**147** (a) Classify this bony defect.
(b) How can such a defect be detected and diagnosed?
(c) Outline at least 3 treatment options for this type of defect.

**148** What are the significant age-related changes in the periodontal tissues and how do they affect treatment?

**149** The metalwork for these 4 anterior crown restorations is being tried in place. What errors are in the process of being made in the construction of these anterior crown restorations?

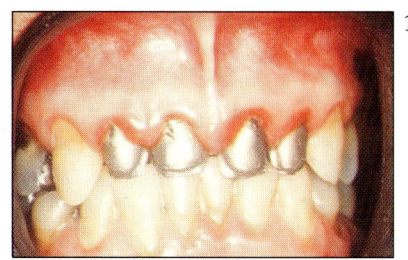

**149**

**150** This 20-year-old male presented with bilateral periocoronitis and both petechiae and ulceration of the palate. He is found to exhibit bilateral cervical lymphadenopathy, fever and malaise.
(a) What is the likely diagnosis?
(b) What tests would you carry out?
(c) What treatment would you carry out?

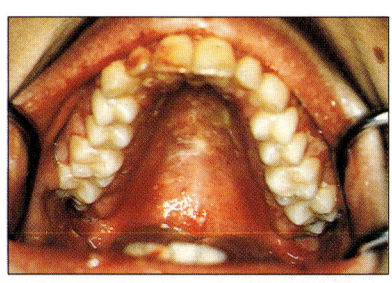

**150**

**151** This 12-year-old male patient who is undergoing orthodontic treatment has become aware of the painless lump on his gum between 32 and 31 over the last 3 months. What is the likely diagnosis and appropriate treatment? What other dental abnormality is present?

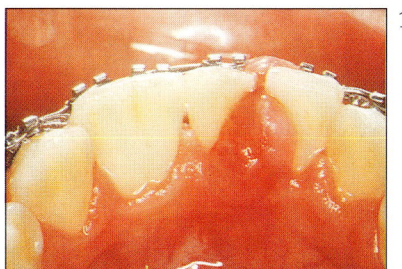

**151**

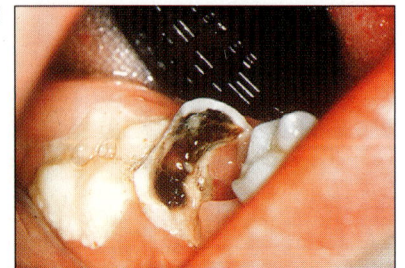

**152** This lower right first permanent molar in a 12-year-old requires extraction.
(a) What are the consequences of the loss of this tooth?
(b) Which other teeth must be taken into consideration?
(c) What is the optimal time for the enforced loss of first permanent molars?

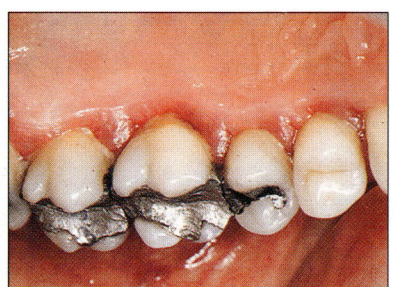

**153** This patient has undergone a course of scaling and plaque control but why does inflammation persist?

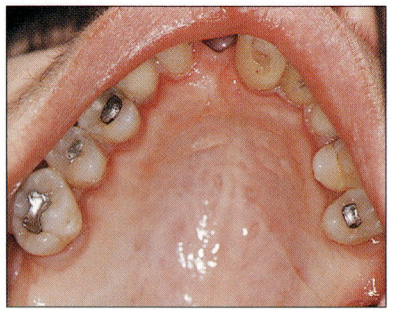

**154** This patient has worn an acrylic partial denture replacing 17, 11, and 26 for 2 years. There is inflammation around the necks of all the teeth, together with some gingival hyperplasia. How may this have arisen and how should it be corrected?

**155** (a) Name the device illustrated in this case of treated periodontal disease.
(b) What are the indications for its use?
(c) How is it retained?
(d) Which materials can be used for its construction?

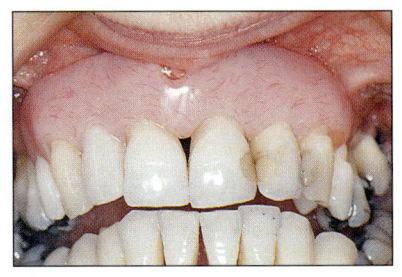

**156** What is this instrument and is it of any benefit to the patient using it?

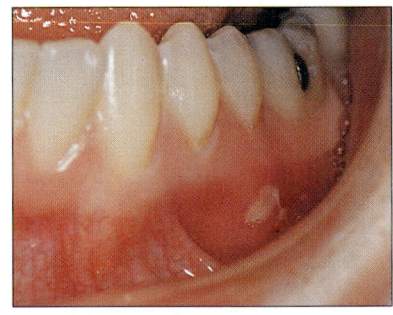

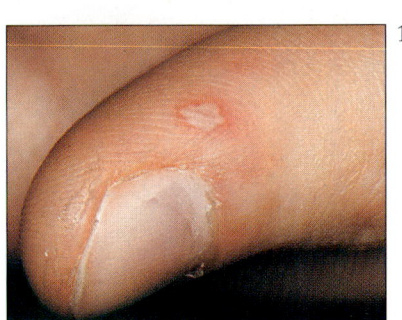

**157** This patient has oral ulcers, each surrounded with a red, inflammatory halo, and gives a history of headache and sore mouth. Further examination reveals vesicular lesions on the lateral aspects of the fingers (**157B**) and the toes.
(a) What is the probable diagnosis of this condition?
(b) What is the causative agent?
(c) To which group of viruses does it belong?
(d) From what types of clinical samples may the virus be isolated?
(e) Is there any specific treatment?

**158**

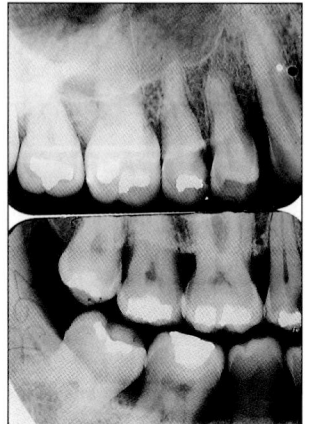

**158** The picture shows two views of the bone levels around a patient's upper molar teeth.
(a) What technique is shown in the upper radiograph and why is it unsuitable for periodontal diagnosis?
(b) Which views are acceptable for recording accurately the bone levels around upper molar teeth?

**159**

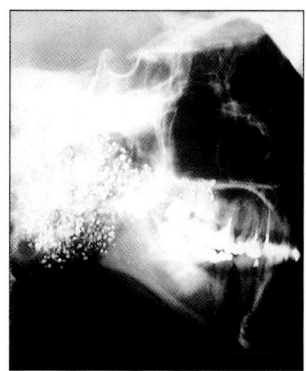

**159** This sialogram with contrast shows the classical 'snow storm' appearance that arises in sialadenitis associated with 'Sjögrens syndrome'.
(a) Define the terms 'primary Sjögrens syndrome' and 'secondary Sjögrens syndrome'.
(b) In diagnosing Sjögrens syndrome what special investigations are useful to perform and why?
(c) How should the periodontium be managed in such cases?

**160**

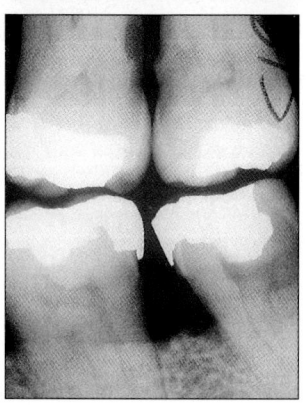

**160** This radiograph shows moderate bone loss in a patient aged 60 years. What is the most likely diagnosis and what other types of periodontitis are there?

**161** The mother of this 7-year-old boy consults you because of what she considers to be the abnormal length of 31 and is worried that it may have recession which may lead to its loss. What advice would you give?

161

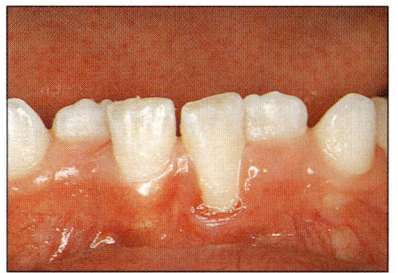

**162** This stain could not be removed with either powered or hand scalers. How was it caused?

162

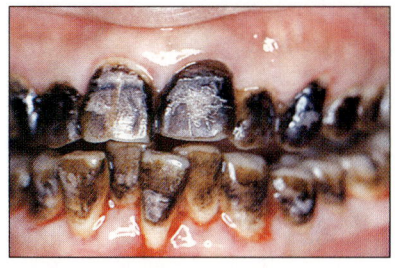

**163** This patient presents in your surgery complaining about the swollen and tender gum associated with 22. The crown restoration was cemented 2 weeks previously.
(a) What is the differential diagnosis?
(b) How should this problem be managed?

163

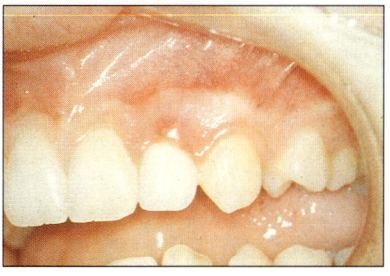

**164** (a) What are the main microscopic features typically seen in Gram-stained smears of debris scraped from ulcers of patients with acute necrotising ulcerative gingivitis (ANUG)?
(b) Which are the predominant types of micro-organisms seen in wet preparations of dental plaque material from ANUG patients when viewed by dark-field or phase-contrast microscopy?
(c) Which micro-organisms have been recovered in highest numbers in cultures of dental plaque from patients with ANUG?
(d) What systemic antimicrobial agents may be used as part of the treatment for patients with ANUG?

**165**

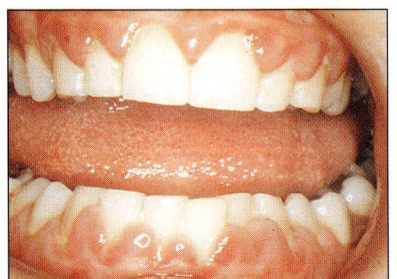

**165** This patient has established chronic gingivitis but is otherwise healthy. List the mechanical cleaning methods that could be used to treat this condition.

**166A**

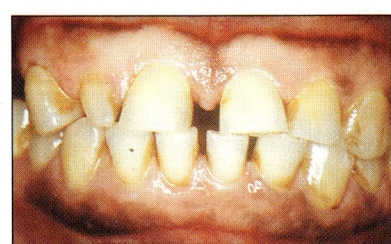

**166** This 45-year-old woman presented complaining of increased spacing between the upper anterior teeth. The teeth present were:

| 18 16 13 12 11 | 21 22 23 28 |
|---|---|
| 48 45 44 43 42 41 | 31 32 33 34 35 36 |

A basic periodontal examination (BPE) revealed $\dfrac{3 \mid 4 \mid 3}{3 \mid 3 \mid 3}$.

**166B**

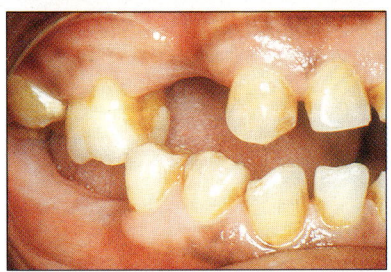

**166A** shows the anterior teeth in the intercuspal position, **166B** the first tooth contact in the retruded arc of closure of the mandible and **166C** the upper and lower right sextants in the intercuspal position.

(a) What are the factors that have led to the tooth migration?

(b) Suggest a provisional treatment plan.

**166C**

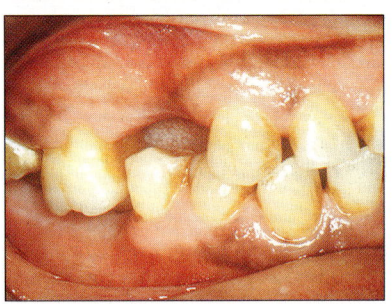

**167** This patient demonstrates a rare condition that is occasionally associated with hypertrichosis.
(a) What is this condition ?
(b) How should the condition be managed ?

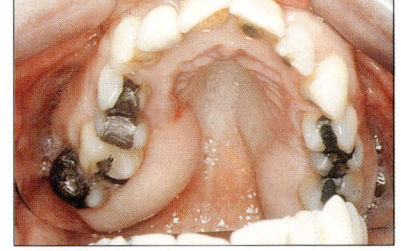
**167**

**168** This patient, aged 24, has had gingival hyperplasia in the lower incisor region for most of his life. The condition did not respond to routine treatment with scaling and oral hygiene instruction and a gingivectomy was carried out 2 months before this photograph was taken. In spite of good plaque control the hyperplasia has returned. Why is this? A radiograph of the affected area is shown in **168B**

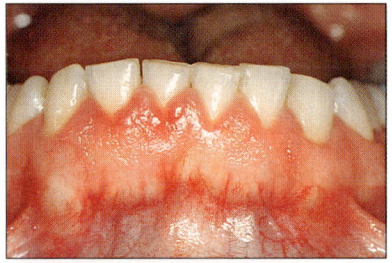
**168A**

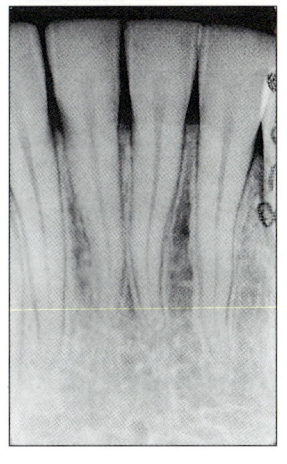
**168B**

**169** Chlorhexidine is both an antimicrobial and a plaque inhibitory agent. What are the considered mechanisms of action of chlorhexidine in these two processes? Given the local side-effects of chlorhexidine, give examples of the proven clinical supragingival uses of this antiseptic.

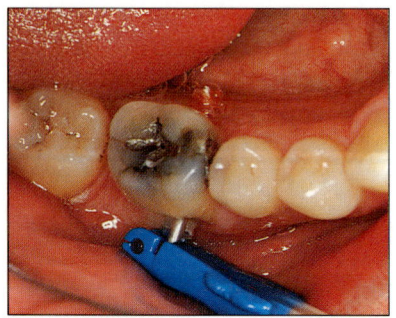

**170** This illustration shows the result of treatment for a grade 3 furcation involvement of tooth 46. What treatment options exist for grade 1, 2 and 3 furcations?

**171**

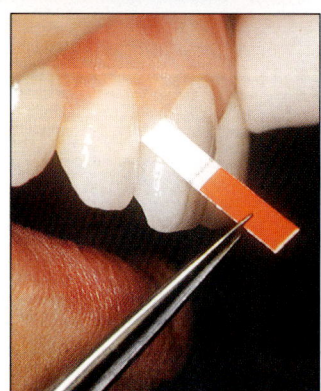

**171** This picture demonstrates gingival crevicular fluid (GCF) sampling using a filter paper strip. This is a commonly used technique prior to analysing the fluid for markers of periodontal disease activity.
(a) What is gingival crevicular fluid and what is its origin?
(b) What are the other common sources of potential markers of periodontal disease activity?
(c) Over what period of time should GCF be sampled prior to analysis, when using filter papers or microcapillary tubes?

**172**

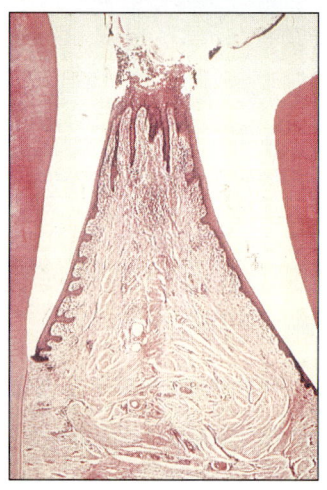

**172** This is a mesio-distal section through the interdental papilla between two molar teeth. What features (not necessarily all determinable in this histological section) might lead you to a diagnosis of:
(a) An initial lesion of gingivitis?
(b) An early lesion of gingivitis?

**173** This is a mesio-distal section through the interdental gingiva between two molar teeth in a subject with an establised lesion of gingivitis (see **172**). What are the histological features of the established lesion of gingivitis?

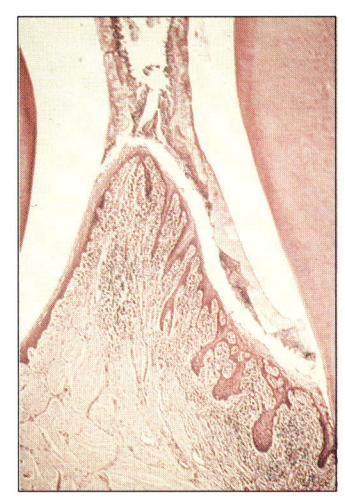

173

**174** This patient has adult periodontitis with a particularly advanced lesion distal to 21. What are the histological features of the advanced lesion? (Features of the initial, early and established lesions have been dealt with in **172** and **173**.)

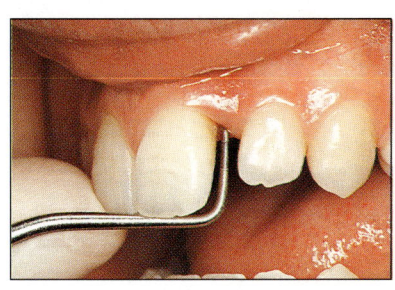

174

**175** What is the name for this type of brush and what is it used for? Name other types of oral hygiene aids designed for the same purpose as this brush. Why are such devices required? How may such devices be detrimental to gingival tissues?

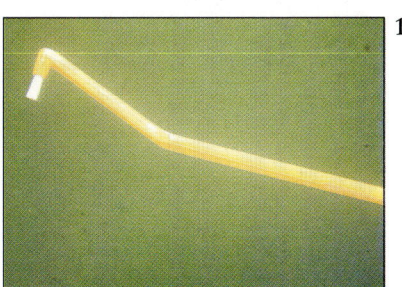

175

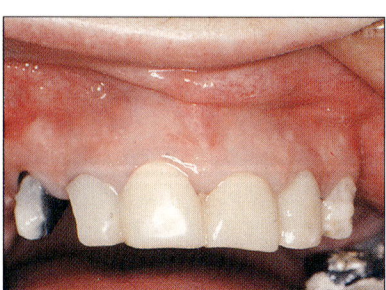
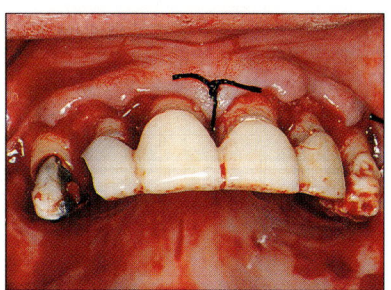

**176** The pictures show apically repositioned flap (ARF) surgery.
(a) What are the 2 main indications for using an apically repositioned flap?
(b) What are the benefits claimed for the ARF procedure when compared with surgical pocket elimination by gingivectomy?
(c) Describe the principal disadvantages of the ARF technique.

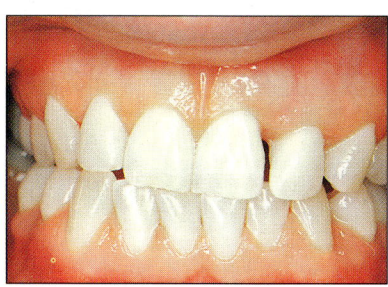
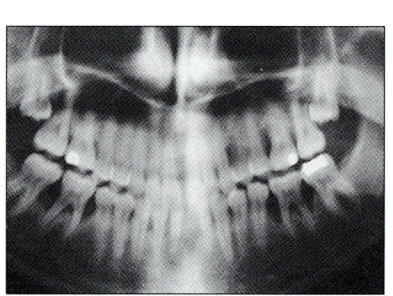

**177** This 14-year-old girl has a space between the upper left central and lateral incisors which has increased in size over the last few months.
Indicate the likely diagnosis, taking into account the radiological findings (**177B**). Outline the possible management of this condition.

**178** What complications are likely to occur in the first post-operative week after gingivectomy?

**179** This patient has abundant deposits both of sub- and supragingival calculus. How do the two differ?

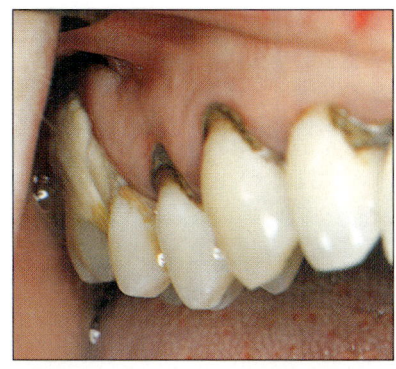

**180** This 2-year-old child was very irritable, had a very sore mouth and was refusing to eat.
(a) What is the likely diagnosis?
(b) With what other conditions might it be confused?
(c) What other signs and symptoms would you expect to observe?
(d) How would you manage this patient?

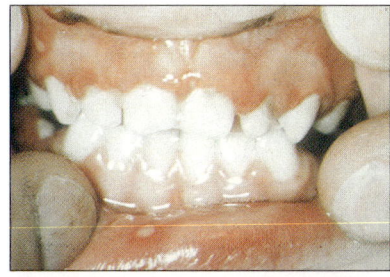

**181** This is the mouth of a 21-year-old patient. His symptoms include feeling generally unwell and a very painful mouth. His temperature is elevated, his gingivae are markedly reddened and his submandibular lymph nodes are enlarged and tender. What is your diagnosis?

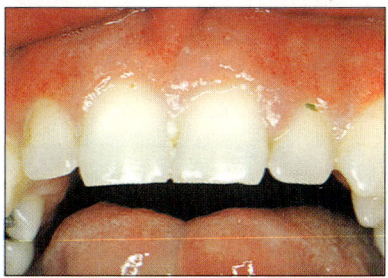

**182** What precautions should be taken in the case of a patient who is taking monoamine-oxidase inhibitors and requires a local anaesthetic for dental treatment?

183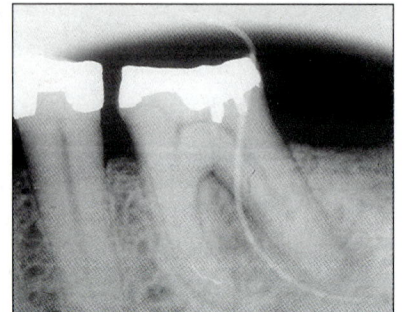

**183** This patient presented with a buccal swelling associated with 36. There was a deep periodontal pocket associated with the distal root of this tooth, and the radiograph shows a guttapercha point placed in this pocket and extending to the apex. Elsewhere in the mouth the periodontal tissues were healthy.
(a) What is your diagnosis?
(b) How would you treat this tooth?

184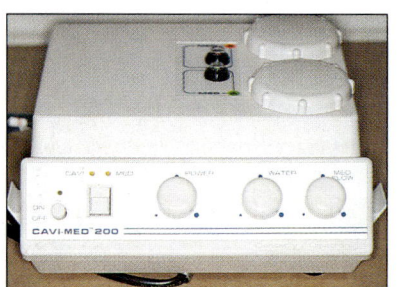

**184** What factors do you have to take into account before this ultrasonic scaler is used on a patient? What are the hazards/complications of its use?

185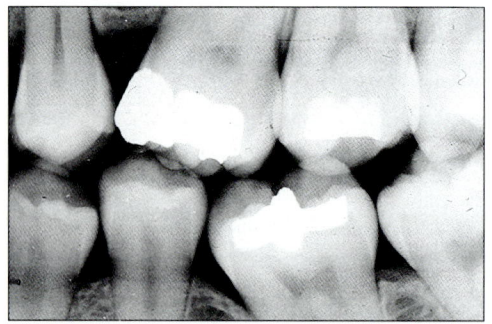

**185** This bitewing radiograph is of a 22-year-old patient. What is the significance of the bone level between the lower second premolar and the molar?

**186** This young female has generalised chronic gingivitis and a few sites of early loss of attachment. In the management of her periodontal conditions what are the actual and/or perceived benefits she might derive from using a mouthwash? In the same context what are the limitations of such mouthwashes?

**186**
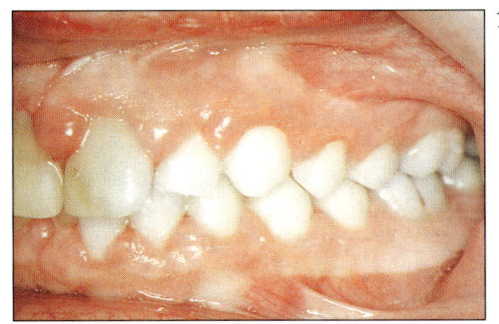

**187** (a) What anatomical feature is contributing to increased probing depth.
(b) List the treatment options.
(c) Describe the surgical options and their relative merits.

**187**
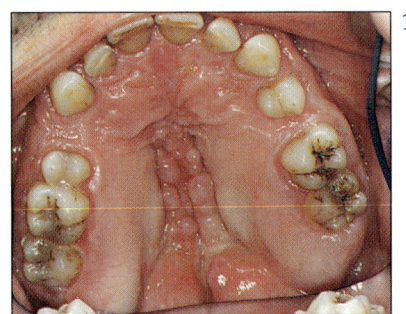

**188** (a) Why is there a deep periodontal pocket around 22?
(b) What is the prognosis for 22?

**188**
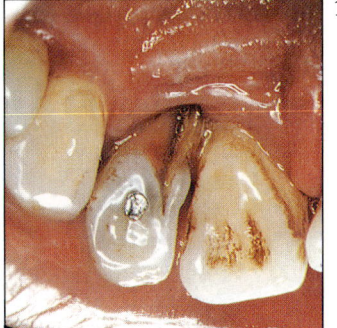

**189**

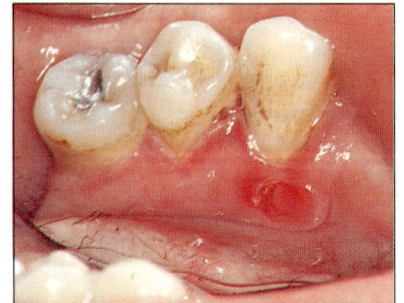

**189** This patient has worn a tissue-borne acrylic partial denture replacing 42–32 for 7 years. He is now complaining of a painful ulcer lingual to 33. There is generalised early periodontitis and oral hygiene is poor. How may his condition be managed?

**190**

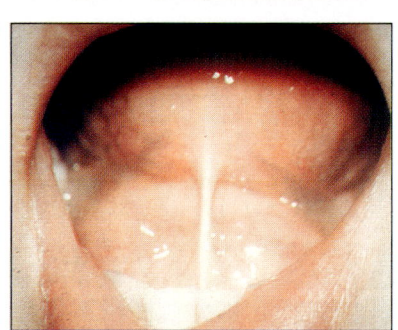

**190** (a) What is this abnormality?
(b) What difficulties may arise as a result of it?
(c) What treatment is required?

**191**

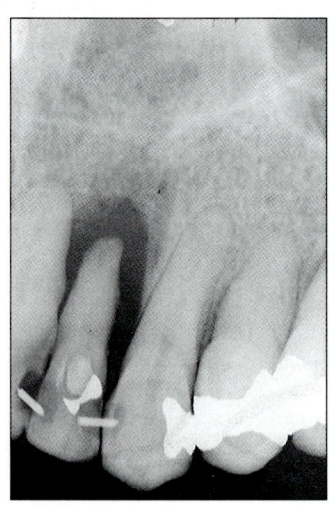

**191** What is the likely sequence of events that led to the appearance of 22 in this radiograph?

**192** This patient presented with a bridge uncemented from abutment 13. The bridge was removed to reveal soft tissue ulceration associated with the proximal gingivae and the fitting surface of the bridge.
(a) What were the causes of this ulceration?
(b) How should this problem be treated?

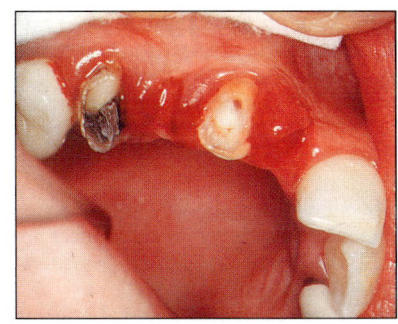

**193** This 12-year-old girl has reddened gums which bleed when she cleans her teeth. Her mother enquires whether 'her age has anything to do with it?' What is the answer?

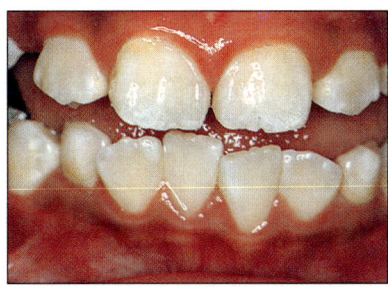

**194** A 40-year-old female patient presents with an acute periodontal abscess associated with a heavily restored upper molar tooth. The treatment plan includes immediate extraction of this tooth under local anaesthesia but the patient gives a history of rheumatic fever and therefore requires antibiotic cover to prevent subsequent development of infective endocarditis.
(a) Assuming that the patient is not allergic to penicillin and has not been treated with penicillin more than once during the previous month, what would be the normally recommended antibiotic prescription for prophylaxis in this case?
(b) If the patient is known to be allergic to penicillin, what alternative antibiotic prophylaxis should be recommended?
(c) In the same situation as described in (a) above, what antibiotic regime would be appropriate if the extraction was to be performed under general anaesthesia?

**195** An adult patient who requires extensive scaling and periodontal surgery gives a medical history of valvular heart disease and is known to have had a previous episode of infective endocarditis. When making a treatment plan for this patient, careful consideration must be given to the need for antibiotic prophylaxis.
(a) Should such patients be treated in general dental practice or is it advisable for them to be referred to hospital?
(b) If the patient described above is not allergic to penicillin and has not received penicillin more than once in the previous month, what prophylaxis would be appropriate to cover dental surgical procedures?
(c) If the patient is allergic to penicillin, what alternative prophylactic antibiotics should be given?
(d) What special features come into consideration when formulating a dental treatment plan for such 'high-risk' patients?

**196**

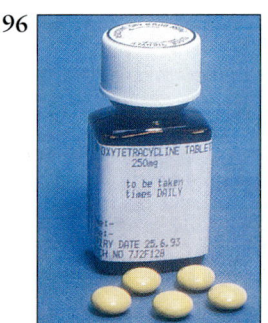

**196** Tetracyclines are useful in the management of early-onset periodontitis. What is the rationale for this, and what unwanted effects are associated with usage of this antimicrobial?

**197A**

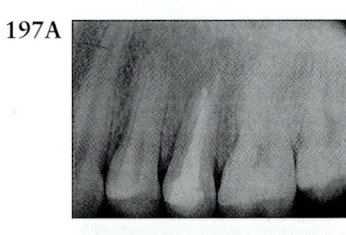

**197B**

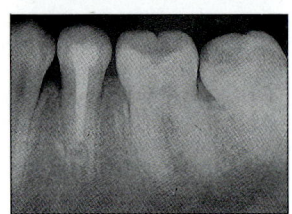

**197** This 14-year-old female had a painful buccal swelling over the 25 which gave a variable response to vitality testing by an electric pulp tester and the application of ethyl chloride. Eventually the tooth was root-filled. A month later the 35 erupted and was associated with a similar lesion.
(a) How could the vitality of these teeth have been confirmed?
(b) If non-vital what is the most likely aetiology of these lesions?

**198** This 30-year-old man has noticed spacing developing between his upper incisors. List the reasons why in this and in other situations upper incisors may migrate.

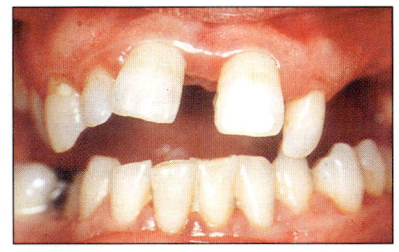
198

**199** A patient presents complaining of the forward migration and lengthening of his upper left central incisor tooth. A periapical radiograph indicates extensive bone loss associated with this tooth. What are the factors which have led to this problem?

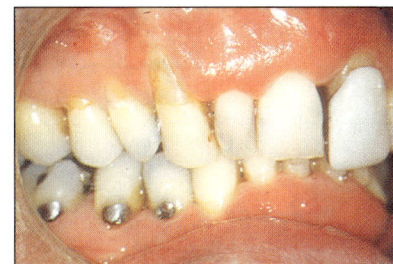
199A

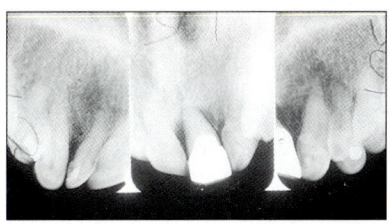
199B

**200** This 17-year-old Afro-Caribbean patient has periodontal pocketing in the incisor and first molar areas.
(a) What is the likely diagnosis?
(b) What antibiotic regimes could be used for this condition?
(c) What precautions should be taken before prescribing antibiotics for this patient?

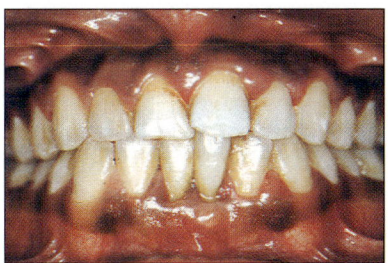
200

**201**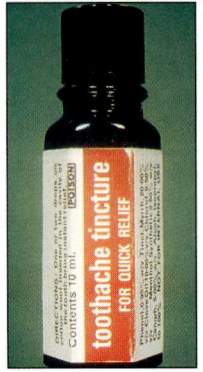

**201** What are the likely constituents of this toothache tincture? What is its supposed mode of action and which constituent is likely to cause damage if it is applied directly to the gum?

**202** What drugs, used in dentistry, can cause an anaphylactic reaction? What are the signs and symptoms of such a reaction and how should the patient be managed?

**203**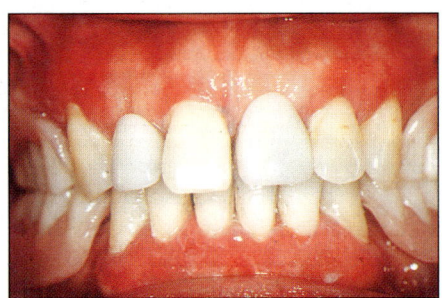

**203** (a) What is the term applied to the clinical picture demonstrated on the gingivae of this middle aged female patient? (b) What are the possible underlying medical conditions that may give rise to this presentation? (c) This patient had condition (iv)(see Answer section). What are the characteristic histological features of this condition?

**204** What are the various mechanisms which may account for drug-induced gingival overgrowth?

**205** This 23-year-old male patient was referred to a periodontist by his general dental practitioner for treatment of his swollen gingiva. The patient has a history of epilepsy. What is the likely cause of the gingival enlargement and how would you manage the case?

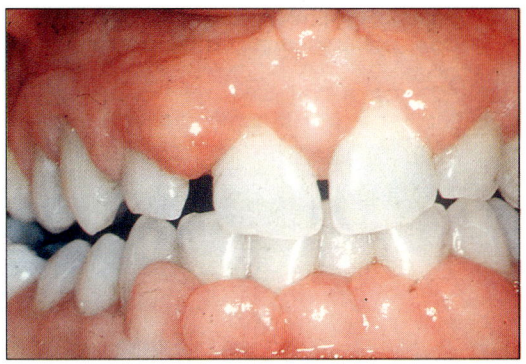

**205**

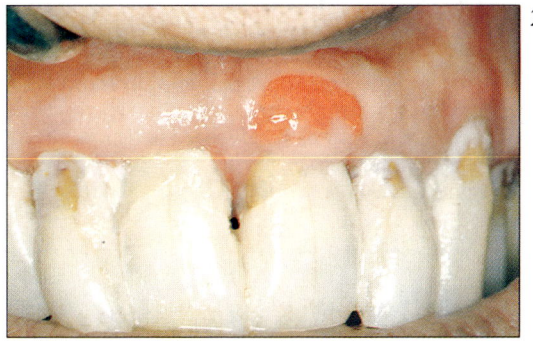

**206**

**206** The picture shows a patient with a lateral periodontal abscess.
(a) Are the causative micro-organisms likely to be of exogenous or endogenous origin?
(b) Are there any known local factors in the mouth which can precipitate the formation of such abscesses?
(c) Which micro-organisms are commonly present in lateral periodontal abscesses?
(d) What are the indications for systemic antibiotic treatment in patients with a periodontal abscess?

**207** What are the causes of xerostomia? What are the dental implications and how can this condition be managed?

**208** What are the problems associated with carrying out periodontal treatment on patients taking systemic corticosteroids?

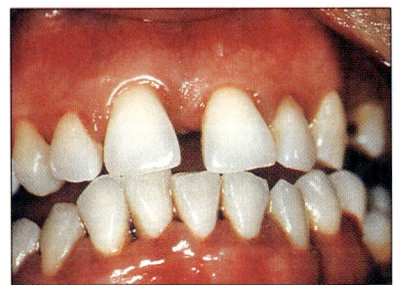

**209** This 38-year-old patient attended with the complaint that her upper incisors, which were once well-aligned, had been drifting over the course of the previous year. Examination reveals that there is generalised periodontitis with basic periodontal examination (BPE) scores of:

$$\frac{3|4|3}{3|3|3}.$$

Oral hygiene is moderate with plaque scores of 60%. 36 was extracted seven years ago, 26 has over-erupted and occlusal examination reveals that there is a marked occlusal interference between 26 and 35 on closure between the retruded axis arc and the intercuspal positions. In addition, 11 has escaped the control of the lower lip at rest. X-ray examination shows generalised bone loss in the upper incisor region, with more advanced bone loss affecting 11.

The patient requests that her appearance be restored to its former state. Assuming that 11 is saveable, suggest a treatment plan appropriate for this patient.

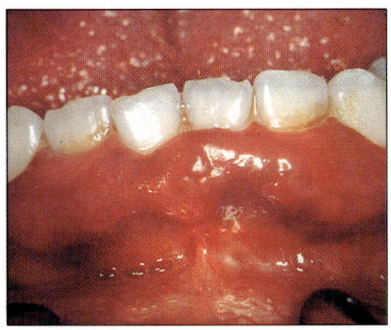

**210** This photograph demonstrates mild *generalised* gingival enlargement. List the possible causes of gingival enlargement/overgrowth.

**211** This 50-year-old male has generalised gingival recession. What anatomical factors may predispose to localised or generalised gingival recession and what aetiological factors may induce the recession? What are the clinical implications of gingival recession?

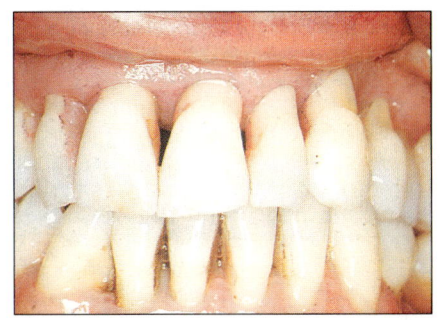

**211**

**212** A 30-year-old woman presented with a long-standing hyperplastic gingival condition. What is the likely diagnosis and how would you confirm this? What treatment would you advise?

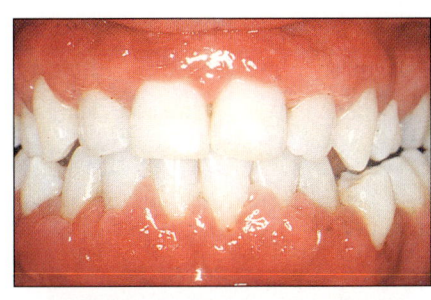

**212**

**213** This female patient, aged 48, has had a number of lateral periodontal abscesses over the last 6 months. She has localised areas of advanced bone loss, one of which distal to 33 was root planed 2 weeks before this photograph was taken. Following the root planing she complained of pain and swelling in the area, as well as in relation to 45, which has been root planed at the same time. What is the likely diagnosis and how should the patient be managed?

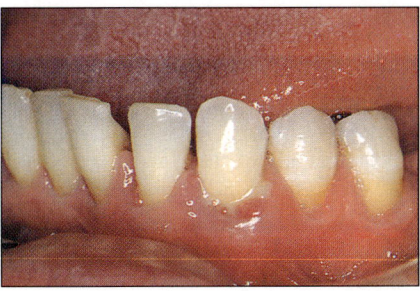

**213**

**214** Dental plaque forms rapidly on clean tooth surfaces in the mouth and is known to develop and mature over a period of time. Thus it is possible to describe plaque at different stages of development as 'early' and 'mature' or 'late' or 'established' plaque.

(a) Starting with a completely clean, polished surface, what process may precede or accompany bacterial deposition and colonisation?

(b) Early bacterial colonisers have a particular ability to attach to the tooth surface during plaque formation. Which particular types of micro-organisms are associated with early plaque?

(c) Following initial plaque formation, what are the main changes that can be observed as plaque develops over a period of 7–10 days?

(d) What are the main characteristics of 'mature' dental plaque?

**215**

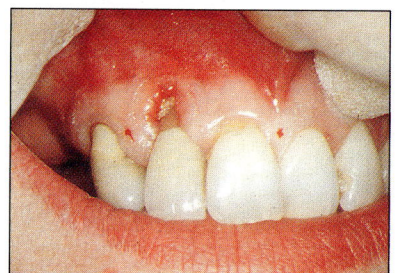

**215** This patient attends your surgery as an emergency, complaining of pain 1 week after root canal treatment of the 12. A sequestrum is seen presenting at the gingival margin buccally. How should this clinical problem be investigated?

**216** Define the following terms used in periodontology:

(a) 'Reattachment'.

(b 'New attachment'.

(c) 'Repair'.

(d) 'Regeneration'.

(e) What is the name given to the process by which new fibrous tissue attachment to a treated root surface is encouraged?

**217**

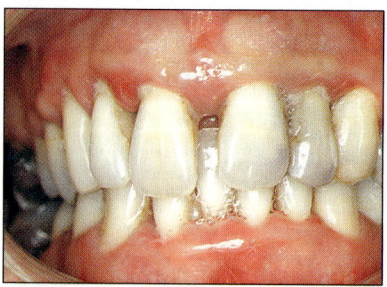

**217** This 40-year-old patient has basic periodontal examination (BPE) scores of 4 in all sextants. Radiographs show generalised moderately advanced bone loss throughout the mouth. You make a diagnosis of adult periodontitis. Outline a suitable treatment plan.

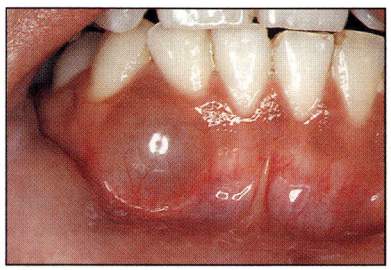

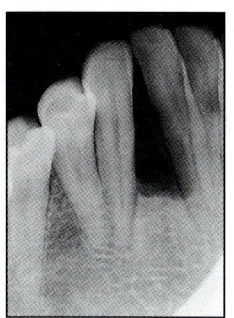

**218** This 24-year-old male patient has fluctuant swelling between 44 and 43, both of which are vital. He has been aware of the swelling for two months. A radiograph (**218B**) reveals extensive loss of bone. What is the likely diagnosis and what is the appropriate treatment?

**219** What are the problems of prescribing drugs used in dentistry to pregnant women?

**220** Medium-to-long term anticoagulant therapy is frequently prescribed for patients who are at risk of suffering a thromboembolic episode. Does this affect the periodontal condition to an appreciable extent or the treatment offered?

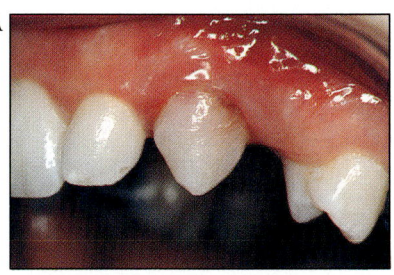

**221** This 21-year-old female patient was complaining of discharge from the buccal surface of 23 which was discoloured and had been transplanted from the palate 8 years previously. A deep pocket was present and the radiograph is shown in **221B**.
(a) What is the lesion and what has caused it?
(b) What could have been done at the time of the transplantation which would have made the occurrence less likely?
(c) What would be an appropriate treatment plan?

**222**  The community peridontal index of treatment needs (CPITN) is endorsed by the World Health Organisation and the Federation Dentaire Internationale for periodontal screening, but was not specifically intended for dental practice. It has been adopted for such use in Britain by the British Society of Periodontology as the 'basic periodontal examination' (BPE), and in the United States by the American Dental Association and the American Academy of Periodontology as 'periodontal screening and recording' (PSR). In both systems the mouth is examined in sextants and the periodontal tissues examined with a WHO probe. Only the highest score is recorded for each sextant. The codes used are the same:

| | |
|---|---|
| 0 = Health | No active treatment. |
| 1 = Bleeding on probing | Removal of plaque, plus oral hygiene instruction (OHI) |
| 2 = Calculus or overhang | OHI plus scaling and correction of margins. |
| 3 = Coloured band partially obscured. | ? |
| 4 = Coloured band completely obscured | ? |

The procedures involved following scores of 3 and 4 differ for the BPE and the PSR. What are these differences?

**223**  A patient with a badly neglected mouth and an ill-fitting partial upper denture (**223A**) attended for dental treatment. On removal of the acrylic appliance, most of the denture-bearing area was found to be red and inflamed (**223B**).
(a) What type of micro-organism is associated with this disorder?
(b) What name or names have been given to this particular clinical manifestation of infection?
(c) How can diagnosis be confirmed in the laboratory?
(d) What underlying conditions may predispose to oral infections with this particular micro-organism?
(e) How should this condition be treated?

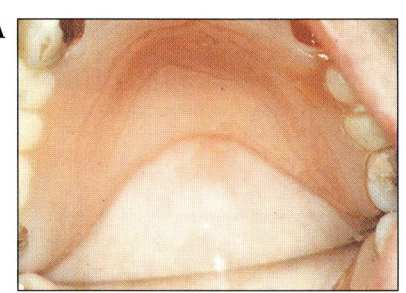

223B

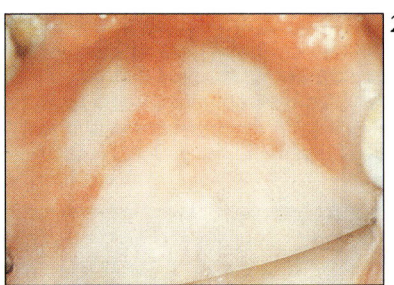

**224** The patient in **224A** presented with extensive swelling and redness of one side of the face and several discharging sinuses. A sample of pus from one of the sinuses was used to prepare the Gram-stained smear shown in **224B**.

(a) What is the diagnosis of this condition?

(b) Which micro-organism is the most common aetiological agent in this infection? Is it normally isolated in pure culture, or in association with other organisms?

(c) When attempting to diagnose this condition, what should be looked for in samples of pus?

(d) What is the most likely source of the causative micro-organisms?

(e) Does this condition occur in other parts of the body?

(f) How should it be treated?

**224A**

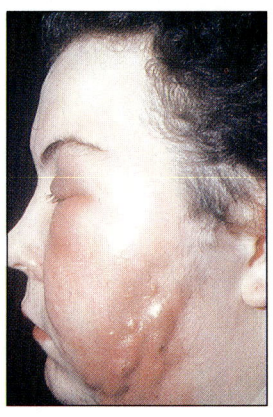

**224B**

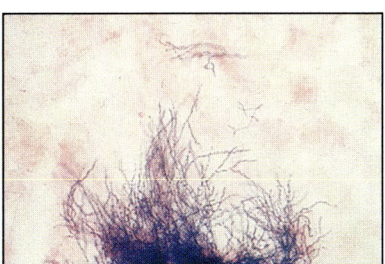

**225**  A 22-year-old female patient presented with a firm, painless swelling of the interdental papilla between 33 and 34 (**225A**), which had been present for about a year. Both teeth were vital to pulp testing and there were no periodontal pockets. A radiograph (**225B**) revealed a radiolucency between the two teeth.
(a) What is the differential diagnosis?
(b) How might the patient be managed?

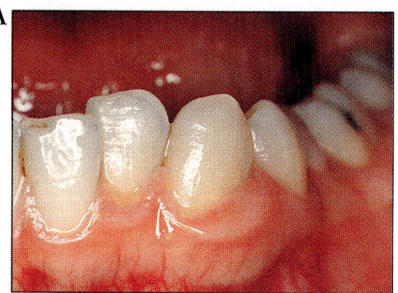

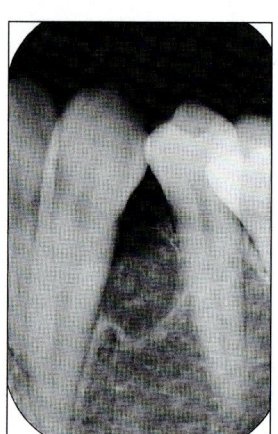

# ANSWERS

**1** The cause of the lesion is toothbrush trauma. It is unlikely to be acute leukaemia since the patient looked well, gave no history of feeling lethargic and the mouth elsewhere is in good health. Leukaemic ulcers rarely have a bleeding surface—the bleeding in acute leukaemia is usually a persistent slight ooze from a vessel within a periodontal pocket. A clue to the traumatic nature of the ulcers is that they are buccal to the canine/first premolar teeth which are prominent in the arch and are commonly traumatised by the toothbrush.

A useful diagnostic test for ulceration which is obviously painful but which is suspected of being self-inflicted is to apply disclosing solution to the area. It is surprising how often the tooth surface will be found to be completely clean—showing that the patient has cleaned the tooth effectively in spite of the discomfort that this would obviously cause.

In this case, the patient was advised to cease all toothbrushing for 2 weeks but to use a chlorhexidine mouthwash instead. The lesion healed uneventfully.

**2** (a) (i) Failure of patient to take medication. (ii) Incorrect initial diagnosis. (iii) Underlying systemic disorder (e.g. leukaemia). (iv) Secondary infection of ulcers by organisms resistant to metronidazole, in a patient whose resistance to infection is impaired. (b) Recheck the history and compliance with the instructions about medication. Take a smear for cytology, a swab for culture and sensitivity and alter the prescription to a broad spectrum antibiotic (immediately and modify if necessary when the sensitivity results are available). Perform a full haematological screen, give dietary advice and review after a week. The gingival tissues are shown 21 days after presentation (**2B**). The student admitted to a poor diet and extreme stress induced by final examinations. The ulcers healed following improved diet and penicillin V therapy.

**3** (a) The microflora associated with LJP are predominantly Gram-negative rods. These include: *Actinobacillus actinomycetemcomitans* (*Aa*);*Capnocytophaga* species; *Eikenella corrodens*. Of these, the strongest evidence of association has been reported for *Aa*. (b) In addition to conventional plaque control measures, treatment with a course of tetracycline has been shown to be effective in many cases and may reduce the risk of recurrence. (c) Several different species have been described in association with RPP and, once again, these are mainly Gram-negative. Prominent among the putative pathogens are: *Actinobacillus actinomycetemcomitans; Porphyromonas gingivalis* (*Pg*) (formerly *Bacteriodes gingivalis*); *Prevotella intermedia* (formerly *Bacteriodes intermedius*); 'corroding bacteria'; spirochaetes (*Treponema* species).

(d) Several virulence factors have been described, particularly for *Aa* and *Pg*, including:
   *Aa*—Leucotoxin, collagenase, endotoxin, epitheliotoxin, fibroblast inhibitory factor, bone resorption inducing factor.
   *Pg*—Typsin-like activity, collagenase, fibrinolysin, other proteases, phospholipase, phosphatases, endotoxin, $H_2S$, $NH_3$, fatty acids.

**4** (a) Rapidly progressive periodontitis.
(b) There is evidence of severe and rapid bone destruction after which the destructive process may dramatically slow down or spontaneously cease. The gingival tissue during the active phase may exhibit marginal proliferation and acute inflammation whereas in the quiescent phase the gingivae may appear free of inflammation. There is evidence of functional defects in monocytes and leucocytes.
(c) Patients appear to respond well to closed/open curettage combined with a course of antibiotics (3-week course of oxytetracycline—250mg 4 times daily) and meticulous hygiene.

**5** The logical answer would be to state that these local anatomical factors may cause problems with oral hygiene. However, there is no evidence to support this; indeed studies suggest that such anomalies do not influence gingival health to any meaningful extent. Thus, nothing should be done to correct such anatomical anomalies. Mucogingival surgical techniques may bring about a more usual anatomical appearance but this presupposes they will also influence cleaning behaviour which is the more fundamental variable in plaque control practices. Sometimes toothbrushing may be difficult and lead to abrasion and soreness of the fraenum. In these circumstances a frenectomy and free gingival graft may be helpful.

**6** This is a delayed (Type IV) hypersensitivity reaction to the temporary crown material. In this case, the temporary crown was made from Scutan, an ethylene amine. The response is usually due to the unpolymerised material. The Scutan crown should be removed and replaced with a new temporary one made from acrylic resin.

**7** No, there are ample local factors to explain the periodontal disease in this case. On the basis of epidemiological studies, there is evidence that periodontal diseases are more prevalent in patients with uncontrolled diabetes. However, the question should be asked, 'Why is the diabetes uncontrolled?'. Is it because many such patients are not managing their diet and drug regime as they should? If so perhaps they are not looking after their plaque control either. Diabetics are particularly prone to periodontal abscesses and loss of attachment. On the other hand even severely affected diabetics, provided that they are well controlled, may have good periodontal health, so local and individual factors are more important than the diabetes *per se*.

**8** (a) The condition is scleroderma and the signs shown in the photograph are thinning of the lips and tightening of the skin around the mouth causing restricted opening (microstomia), gross gingival recession and gross deformity of the hands (sclerodactyly). The skin takes on an ivory, waxy appearance.
(b) The periodontal ligament is widened in scleroderma with gradual obliteration of the lamina dura, and there may be associated Sjögren's disease. Periodontal disease may progress rather rapidly because of the xerostomia, the microstomia, advanced gingival recession and the sclerodactyly which makes holding a toothbrush very difficult. There is progressive induration of the skin with fixation of the epidermis to the subcutaneous tissues.

(c) Oral hygiene needs to be maintained at a high level. Use of an electric toothbrush or modification of a conventional toothbrush and interdental brush by providing them with thick overhandles, more easily held and manipulated, is often useful. The use of a 0·2% chlorhexidine mouthwash or a 0·1% solution delivered by an oral irrigator will keep plaque levels low. Exercises are said to prevent worsening of the microstomia. If extraction of the posterior teeth seems likely to be necessary, they should be removed before undue difficulty of access makes the procedure difficult. Patients with scleroderma benefit from seeing a hygienist at intervals of 2 to 3 months.

**9** (a) (i) Chronic adult periodontitis with occlusal trauma. (ii) Parafunction, probably nocturnal bruxing.
(b) (i) Plaque control using an interspace brush and dental tape. (ii) An occlusal appliance to protect the teeth and soft tissues. A Michigan design would be appropriate enclosing buccal cusps and incisal edges of the maxillary teeth. (iii) Study casts to monitor any tooth migration or further tooth wear.

**10** Disorders of the immune system can be considered either primary or secondary. The primary disorders are usually genetically determined and rare. These include hypogamma-globulinaemia, Di George syndrome and IgA deficiency. Patients with primary immuno-deficiencies experience reduced gingival inflammation, but an increased propensity to periodontal breakdown. However, such cases are extremely rare and it is difficult to draw any conclusions about the effects of such immunodeficiencies on the periodontium.

The secondary immunodeficiencies can be caused by disease or drug therapy. Diseases associated with secondary immunodeficiencies include AIDS, diabetes mellitus, sarcoidosis, sickle-cell disease, renal disease and plasma cell dyscrasia. Immunosuppressant drugs include corticosteroids, azathioprine and cyclosporin. Patients on these drugs appear to be afforded some degree of protection against periodontal breakdown. These findings would suggest that activation of a viable and fully functional system is important in the patho-genesis of such breakdown.

**11** (a) Acute necrotising ulcerative gingivitis (ANUG). A characteristic feature of ANUG is the destruction of interdental papillae. In this case, the papillae between 12 and 11 and between 21 and 22 show advanced destruction while that between 11 and 21 shows destruction at an earlier stage.
(b) The recession labial to 11 could be treated non-surgically or surgically. Non-surgical treatment would involve scaling and plaque control, advice on stopping smoking, followed by root planing if inflammation persisted. When the periodontal condition is stable, a gingival veneer (gum slip) could be made in acrylic resin. This should be worn for social occasions only and the patient should not wear it while asleep.

**12** (a) The most likely reason for lack of success of the apicectomy was failure to secure an effective apical seal. In addition it would appear that far more root has been removed than was necessary.
(b) Possible treatment options for the patient are: (i) Extraction of the tooth and eventual replacement by a bridge. (ii) Extraction followed by an implant. In this case, with the loss of labial bone it is likely that postextraction resorption would leave too slender an alveolus to accommodate an implant without ridge augmentation by guided tissue regeneration. (iii) Reseal the apex of 21 and attempt coverage of the root surface by a laterally or coronally repositioned flap.

Of these possibilities, (iii) was chosen. A three-sided labial flap was raised from the mesial of 21 to 23. The bone defect was curetted and the root surface cleaned and planed. A cavity was cut in the root face and resealed with amalgam. The flap was trimmed mesially to remove sufficient tissue for the interdental papilla that originally lay between 21 and 22 to augment what remained of the papilla between 11 and 21, and the tissue that originally formed the papilla between 22 and 23 became the new papilla between 21 and 22, leaving a triangular area of exposed bone between 22 and 23. A periosteal release incision was necessary high on the deep surface of the flap to give it sufficient mobility to be placed where required.

The wound was sutured and dressed. Healing was satisfactory, although some shrinkage of the flap did occur and a little root surface remained exposed. This was corrected by tooth preparation for a new crown which had a cervical margin of pink porcelain. Follow-up radiographs showed successful apical healing and the appearance was satisfactory 10 years later (**12C**).

**13** (a) Repaired bilateral cleft of alveolus, hard and soft palate.
(b) (i) Residual oro-nasal fistula after reparative surgery. (ii) Collapse of the maxilla due to scar tissue. (iii) Orthodontic problems, poor occlusion. (iv) Difficulty carrying out adequate oral hygiene, particularly in maxillary incisor region. (v) Hypodontia in the line of the cleft. (vi) Enamel hypoplasia.
(c) The incidence of all clefts is approximately 1 in 600, but there are considerable racial differences. Cleft lip with or without involvement of the alveolus occurs in 25% of cases and is more common in males. Unilateral and bilateral clefts of lip and palate are found in 40% and 10% of cases respectively. Cleft palate is found in about 25% of cases.

**14** (i) Radiation burns of skin if dosage is poorly controlled.
(ii) Radiation mucositis, damage to the oral mucosa in the first 2 to 3 weeks after treatment. It presents with a yellow-white surface membrane after 7 days. This is followed by surface shedding and erythema, prior to recovery.
(iii) Salivary gland damage and fibrosis, leading to xerostomia.
(iv) Fibrosis/ankylosis of the temporomandibular joint (TMJ).
(v) Disruption of cartilagenous growth centres, e.g. TMJ cartilage leading to facial growth disorders and asymmetry.
(vi) Pulpal necrosis induced directly by the radiation.
(vii) Predisposition to cervical caries and periodontal disease is an indirect effect of xerostomia.
(viii) Aseptic necrosis of bone due to direct damage to osteocytes and also indirectly as a result of endarteritis obliterans, which eliminates feeding blood vessels within the bone. The residual bone is brittle and prone to infection.
(ix) Radiation-induced osteomyelitis. This is a late complication and an indirect effect involving the bone marrow space. There is a tendency towards sequestrum formation and occasionally pathological fractures occur.
(x) Predisposition to malignancy due to the mutagenic effects upon certain cells. This is a very late-stage complication.

The periodontal tissues should be managed by reducing plaque build-up, particularly at the cervical margins of teeth. This should begin before radiotherapy. Oral hygiene instruction is essential along with fluoride supplements to reduce the likelihood of cervical caries and dietary analysis and advice. The use of artificial saliva may help with xerostomia and a regular maintenance programme should be adopted.

**15** The type of periodontal surgery least likely to cause significant recession is a replaced flap approached by an intracrevicular rather than an inverse-bevel incision. However, in the upper anterior region of the mouth the bone loss is usually palatal and interproximal with the labial bone remaining intact. This can easily be ascertained by probing before surgery. If the labial bone is intact, a palatal flap only should be raised using an intracrevicular incision which should sever the interdental papillae on the palatal side of the contact points. The flap should be reflected to disclose the bone margins and no further. Removal of inflammatory tissue, any remaining calculus and infected cementum is achieved from the palatal side. It is not difficult to extend instrumentation as far round towards the labial surface as is necessary. The wound should then be sutured. Postoperative recession should be minimal.

**16** (i) Intensive oral hygiene instruction, with consistent use of disclosing solution/tablets. Special emphasis on sulcular brushing and use of interspace brushes. No one toothbrush design is most effective for all patients and every patient requires assessment and advice on an individual basis. Obviously, if a high standard of oral hygiene cannot be attained and maintained, then the patient should not be undergoing orthodontic treatment. (ii) Use of a well-formulated fluoride toothpaste. (iii) Dietary advice. (iv) Topical fluoride therapy before the bands and brackets are connected. (v) Use of a daily 0·05% neutral sodium fluoride mouthrinse.

**17** (a) Shingles (zoster). This takes the form of a localised eruption, usually unilateral and confined to one dermatome.
(b) Varicella–zoster virus (VZV): the same virus that causes chickenpox in children. The condition is due to reactivation of the virus, which has remained latent following an earlier clinical or subclinical infection with VZV.
(c) The virus can be demonstrated in vesicle fluid by electron-microscopy. Virus particles may also be seen in biopsy material using immunocytochemical staining methods with monoclonal antibodies. Serological methods may be used to reveal rising titres of antibodies to VZV antigens in acute and convalescent serum samples, or to demonstrate specific IgM antibody at early stages of the infection.
(d) Certain categories of patients are at particularly high risk of serious complications with VZV infection. These include: neonates (within first 3 weeks of life); immunocompromised patients; patients with ophthalmic zoster.
(e) Antiviral chemotherapeutic agents, such as acyclovir, may be used in severe cases and are essential in the treatment of immunocompromised patients with shingles.

**18** The ridge may be locally augmented using a non-resorbable membrane in an effort to regenerate the lost buccal bone and ensure the socket fills with bone. The procedure would involve raising labial and palatal flaps and removing any epithelium and granulation tissue present. The socket could be fenestrated with a small round bur to create bleeding points from adjacent healthy bone. The socket is then packed with a space maintainer, e.g. freeze-dried bone allograft, or a resorbable woven gauze (used for packing bleeding sockets).

The augmentation membrane is adapted over the packed socket to cover the bone margins by 2–3mm. It may be secured at its periphery using small bone screws or cyanoacrylate glue, prior to flap replacement. It is essential to cover the membrane fully and a periosteal relieving incision may be necessary to facilitate this. The membrane is left in place for 6–8 months while bone forms underneath. It is then removed prior to implant placement.

**19** The lesion is a fibroma. A radiograph would be the most obvious first choice for an investigation. The radiograph would inform the clinician of the radio-opacity of adjacent tissues. Given that the radiograph gave negative information, and together with the history and appearance, a fibroma is the most likely diagnosis. Thus, typical of benign tumours, the lesion has been slow growing, has reached considerable proportions and is not inflamed or ulcerated. Additionally and of importance, the tumour has displaced adjacent structures, namely the teeth. These latter features, the consistency and radiolucency of the lesion, together with a lack of radiodensity changes to adjacent structures would tend to rule out most other tumours and epulides such as the fibro-epithelial polyp.
Treatment: excision biopsy and follow-up.

**20** (a) (i) Guttapercha point No 15/20 placed in the buccal sinus with parallax radiographs to confirm the presence and accessibility of the perforation. (ii) Clinical probing of the root canal to judge the size of the perforation and confirm accessibility. (iii) Clinical probing of the gingival sulcus to determine whether a communication exists with the perforation.
(b) (i) If the perforation is small, it might be possible to seal this with vertical condensation of guttapercha from within the root canal. The radiograph suggests a large perforation and in this case a surgical procedure will be required. (ii) A new post core of adequate length, using a post core system that will minimise further tooth destruction will need to be constructed prior to surgery. The post will need to extend well into the apical third of the root of the tooth, beyond the perforation. (iii) Following preparation for the post, leakage of the remaining root filling will need to be assessed. If there is any doubt about the effectiveness of the apical root filling, a retrograde restoration should be placed at the time of surgery. Post cementation should be delayed until the time of surgery. If moisture control is difficult to achieve within the root canal, it should be delayed until after the labial flap has been raised and moisture control achieved. (iv) A full thickness, mucoperiosteal flap should be raised from the gingival margin ensuring that the relieving incisions are kept well away from the region of the perforation and adjacent bone. (v) Bone removal should allow good access to the perforation preferably without removing the bone crest, if this is still present. (vi) Following post cementation and completion of the cement set, any excess cement should be removed, the tooth tissue surrounding the perforation undercut with a small rose head, steel or tungsten carbide bur and a corrosion resistant alloy condensed into the defect. (vii) The flap should be replaced and sutured after root planing, and any exposed root surface covered with the flap. A periodontal pack is unnecessary but a 0·2% chlorhexidine mouthwash should be used for at least one week following surgery. The key to successful treatment of this problem is good access.

**21** The lesion is clearly a form of extreme hyperkeratosis, presumably due to a locally applied tissue irritant and is probably premalignant or malignant. Careful questioning revealed that in contrast to most smokers she indulged in the habit of 'reverse smoking', i.e. having lit the cigarette, she held the burning end in her mouth. This has caused the lesion. The correct treatment is to tell the patient in the strongest possible terms to discontinue the habit of reverse smoking—indeed, to stop smoking altogether. In addition, the lesion should be examined by incisional biopsy as a matter of extreme urgency. Any area which is red rather than white should be included in the biopsy specimen, since areas of redness indicate actively dividing (i.e. malignant) cells, rather than white areas which indicate reactive (i.e. keratin-producing) cells. The patient was given an appointment for the following day for examination by biopsy, but she failed to keep this and the long-term outcome is unknown.

**22** (a) Crescentic bone loss, or angular defects.
(b) It arises from a combination of any form of periodontitis (adult, juvenile or rapidly progressive) with occlusal trauma. This combination is called secondary occlusal trauma, and a parafunctional habit is a characteristic feature. The appearance of the radiograph has been caused by the bone loss palatally, mesially and distally, forming a gutter alongside the tooth thus producing a sharp difference in radiopacity between the lesion and normal bone.
(c) Treatment of secondary occlusal trauma gives priority to resolving the inflammatory component, via scaling and plaque control, followed by root planing. Periodontal flap surgery may also be required. The occlusal element is treated by occlusal analysis, provision of a bite guard and occlusal adjustment as necessary.

**23** The cleft-like lesions on the gingivae near the interdental papillae have been caused by incorrect use of floss. Excessive pressure has been placed by the floss on the gingiva. Occasionally grooves are seen in teeth if the patient uses a see-saw action instead of up and down. It is very important when teaching patients to use floss or tape that they demonstrate how they use it so that faults can be spotted and eliminated. Floss or tape should be used in such a way that the proximal surfaces adjacent to the space are cleaned and the fingers so positioned that proximo-buccal and proximo-lingual surfaces are cleaned as well.

**24** Diagnosis: generalised severe chronic periodontitis.
Clinical findings: (i) attachment loss; (ii) inflammatory signs; (iii) pocket formation; (iv) deposits of supragingival/subgingival calculus; (v) furcation involvement of teeth; (vi) mobility of teeth; (vii) suppuration; (viii) drifting of teeth.

**25** Metronidazole is an effective antimicrobial against anaerobic bacteria which are implicated in periodontal destruction and include *Porphyromonas gingivalis* and *Prevotella intermedius*. The drug has been shown to be of value in the management of advanced adult periodontitis and cases of refractory periodontitis. It is also the treatment of choice of acute necrotising ulcerative gingivitis (ANUG).

Unwanted effects of metronidazole are few. Some patients complain of a metallic taste. There is a significant interaction between metronidazole and alcohol. The drug blocks the enzyme alcohol dehydrogenase, thus alchoholic beverages are not broken down. This can lead to severe hangover effects with nausea and vomiting. Patients must be advised not to drink alcohol while taking this antimicrobial. Animal experiments suggest that metronidazole may be teratogenic; while there is no human data to support this claim, the manufacturers recommend that it is not given during pregnancy.

**26** Before the new denture can be constructed it will be necessary to eliminate the palatal gingival hyperplasia. In this case, the overgrown tissue is too extensive and fibrous to be expected to resolve following conservative measures and it will need to be removed by gingivectomy. This is best done in one visit making sure that all palatal pocketing is completely eliminated. No removal of buccal or labial tissue is necessary. Residual deposits of calculus should then be removed. The existing denture can be used to retain the postoperative dressing which is necessary to prevent tissue regrowth while the wound is healing by epithelisation. This can be achieved very successfully by applying a tissue conditioner to the fitting surface of the denture and trimming away the excess. The patient is shown how to remove the denture twice per day in order to rinse for two minutes with 0.2% chlorhexidine mouthwash. At the same time the denture should be soaked in a hypochlorite denture cleaner. The wound should be inspected at one week and the tissue conditioner replaced. Epithelisation should be complete after approximately 2 weeks when conventional oral hygiene can replace the use of chlorhexidine. Impressions for the new denture can be taken 6 weeks after the gingivectomy. Until then the patient's oral hygiene should be maintained at a high level, the tissue conditioner replaced at 2-week intervals and the denture soaked nightly in a hypochlorite denture cleaner.

**27** Non-vital lateral incisor with a dens in dente. These developmental abnormalities of enamel and dentine often present with pulpal exposure even without tooth preparation. Teeth with such abnormalities are not satisfactory bridge abutments.

This example does merit an attempt to undertake endodontic treatment through the crown restoration although often a surgical approach with retrograde filling of the root canal is the only answer because of the aberrant pulp morphology.

**28** (a) Coe-pak.
(b) Zinc oxide; lorothidol (a fungicide); non-ionising carboxylic (fatty) acid; chlorothymol (bacteriostatic agent).
(c) To protect the wound from accidental trauma and improve patient comfort. To assist in retaining the new position of flap margins and to reduce the amount of dead space by the application of gentle pressure.
(d) (i) Initially soft and sufficiently malleable to allow replacement and optimal adaptation. (ii) Reasonable and variable setting time. (iii) Sufficiently rigid in thin section in the set state to prevent dislodgement. (iv) Have a smooth, non-irritating set surface. (v) Non-toxic. (vi) Bactericidal/fungicidal to discourage plaque formation.
(e) (i) Gypsum and self-curing, plasticised acrylic, e.g. Peripac. (ii) Light-cured polyether urethane dimethacrylate resin, e.g. Barricaid. (iii) Iso-butyl cyanoacrylate tissue adhesive, e.g Bucrylate. (iv) Zinc oxide and eugenol-based dressing.

**29** The history of persistent gingival bleeding and of feeling tired and unwell is strongly suggestive of a blood dyscrasia and steps should be taken to confirm or eliminate this possibility immediately. It is usually most convenient to refer the patient to his medical practitioner as an emergency with a telephone call or a referring letter requesting a 'differential white cell count'. In this case the white cell count was as follows:
'Platelets: $128,000/mm^3$
Leucocytes: $29,700/mm^3$

Differential count:

| | |
|---|---|
| Neutrophils: 3% | Lymphocytes: 4% |
| Eosinophils: – | Monocytes: ⎫ 93% |
| Basophils: – | Abnormal cells ⎭ |

The film shows the presence of many atypical monocytes and promonocytes. Normoblasts and myelocytes are present in the peripheral blood.'

The diagnosis of acute leukaemia was made and confirmed the following day, after a sternal puncture and bone marrow examination. Sadly, the patient died 4 days later from a massive cerebral haemorrhage.

The gingival condition in acute leukaemia can be very variable. Sometimes the gum enlarges and its colour can vary between very pale and redder than normal. The most important oral diagnostic feature in this condition is the persistent gingival bleeding.

30 (a) Antigens: probably the most important of which are lipopolysaccharides. These trigger both immune and inflammatory responses leading to tissue damage. Enzymes: such as collagenase which breaks down collagen, and hyaluronidase responsible for degrading the hyaluronic acid which helps to cement together epithelial cells lining the pocket. A large range of enzymes are released from dental plaque which cause local damage and increase the permeability of the adjacent tissues. Toxic metabolites: Acids such as lactic acid and pyruvic acid cause local damage, while other molecules such as hydrogen sulphide are also damaging. Toxins such as endotoxins released from the cell walls of Gram-negative bacteria. These are powerful antigens as well as causing local damage.
(b) Lipopolysaccharides form part of the cell wall of Gram-negative bacteria and are therefore released after lysis of the organism.
(c) They have wide-ranging effects such as: triggering the immune response; provoking severe inflammation; inhibition of a range of cellular functions; inhibition of connective tissue attachment; and fibroblast cytotoxicity.
(d) Laboratory experiments show that most methods which meticulously abrade the root surface will reduce the endotoxin layer to a very low level. These include root planing, polishing, and extraction with various solvents.

31 The cause of the gingival enlargement is secondary to nifedipine therapy. This drug is a calcium-channel blocker extensively used in the prophylaxis of angina. About 10% of patients who take nifedipine experience gingival overgrowth. Treatment involves surgical excision to restore the gingival contour. This in turn will facilitate plaque control. Recurrence of the gingival overgrowth is likely and it is worthwhile discussing the patient's medication with the physician. Other calcium-channel blockers (i.e. diltiazem, verapamil, amlodipine) all cause gingival overgrowth. Therefore switching the medication to another calcium antagonist may not prevent recurrence. Beta-adrenoceptor blocking drugs, such as atenolol, can also be used in the management of angina. These drugs are not associated with gingival overgrowth.

32 (a) This is produced by habitual picking or scratching at the area. The condition is known as gingivitis artefacta.
(b) Young children, of this age and below, sometimes develop a habit of scratching in areas of irritation. This tends to happen when primary teeth start to become mobile or when permanent teeth commence eruption. When this is discussed with them, they will often give the logical explanation 'it was itchy so I scratched it'! Usually all that is necessary is to point out the problem, counsel the child and parents and treat any local irritation. Occasionally, however, in young children, or in older children, adults and those with learning difficulties, gingivitis artefacta may be an indication of psychiatric problems and psychiatric advice may be required in severe cases.

33 (a) Herpangina.
(b) Coxsackie A virus, especially types 2, 4, 5, 6, 8, 10 and 23.
(c) Occasionally patients with such Coxsackie A infections develop acute parotitis which can be confused with mumps on clinical examination.
(d) Coxsackie A virus may be isolated from the oral lesions, particularly vesicle fluid, and from faeces. An increase in the titre of virus-neutralising antibody in serum can also be demonstrated by examining acute and convalescent blood samples.

**34** The condition is acute generalised periodontitis which is nearly always found in middle-aged patients who have gross calculus deposits and who may, as in this case, be undiagnosed diabetics. In essence the patient has two huge periodontal abscesses involving virtually the whole of each dental arch. Where fluctuant the abscesses should be drained and as much calculus as possible removed, preferably using an ultrasonic scaler which gives a washed field and is quicker and less traumatic than hand instruments. A systemic antibacterial agent should be prescribed. Since the infection is endogenous (i.e. caused by an overgrowth of the patient's own organisms) the bacteria concerned are likely to be Gram-negative anaerobes and either tetracycline (250 mg 4 times daily) or metronidazole (200 mg 3 times daily) both for 1 week are likely to be effective. The patient should be referred to his general medical practitioner who will arrange for the patient to be investigated for diabetes and, if necessary, treated. Removal of deposits should continue until the mouth has healed. When the diabetes is controlled, definitive periodontal treatment can be planned and undertaken.

**35** (a) Both subgingival and supragingival calculus may be seen on these teeth. The supragingival calculus is recognisable because of its light colour and occurs above the gingiva. Clinically the soft texture would also be apparent. This subject also has a line of subgingival calculus present at the enamel-cement junction, in a supragingival location. The most likely scenario is that the patient had active pockets with subgingival calculus formation. Over a period of time, recession occurred leaving the subgingival calculus above the gingiva. Supragingival calculus was subsequently deposited.
(b) Score 3: supragingival calculus covering more than two thirds of the exposed tooth surface or a continuous heavy band of subgingival calculus around the cervical portion of the tooth.
(c) The Retention Index score would also be 3: large cavity, abundance of calculus or grossly insufficient marginal fit of a dental restoration in a supra- or subgingival location. As the description indicates, the Retention Index is unique in that it scores plaque-retaining agents with regard to their relationship to the gingival margin and without regard to the type of factor.

**36** Examination of the child will quickly reveal a vesicular eruption in his mouth, bright red gums and submandibular lymphadenopathy. He has primary herpetic gingivostomatitis which has involved his eczematous lesions producing herpetic eczema. The lesion on his forehead has probably been produced by scratching the skin with a finger infected with the virus by sucking. He is very ill and should be hospitalised without delay. Treatment should consist of systemic acyclovir (200 mg 5 times per day) and adequate hydration must be maintained. No more betamethasone cream should be applied to the eczema since this would accelerate the spread of the virus. The child is in danger of contracting an uncommon but serious complication of herpes simplex infection, herpetic encephalo-meningitis.

**37** (a) Coronally repositioned or advanced flap.
(b) Free gingival or mucosal graft. Used in order to create a 'cosmetic' width of keratinised tissue, although the lighter colour of the grafted mucosa may detract from the final result. The grafting procedure should also ensure sufficient length of tissue to advance the flap without eliminating the adjacent vestibular sulcus.
(c) (i) Citric acid has been applied to exposed roots during surgery in an endeavour to enhance new cementum formation and fibrous attachment to their surfaces. Exposed collagen and dentinal tubules created by the demineralisation process are said to encourage

early cell and fibrous adherence. Results are ambiguous. (ii) Guided tissue regeneration can be successful provided the membrane can be placed apically enough to avoid exposure and sufficient space beneath the membrane can be maintained.

**38** Tooth malalignment is predisposing to plaque retention which, in turn, is the direct cause of the gingivitis. This only occurs when the patient's plaque control is poor. If plaque control is generally poor, there will be inflammation in all areas, whereas when patients are motivated to high standards of oral hygiene, they will usually be able to overcome the difficulties of cleaning those areas where access is a problem.

**39** This photomicrograph shows a large number of dentinal tubules open at the surface and approximately 1 micron in diameter. A hydrodynamic mechanism is generally accepted to explain stimulus transmission across dentine and therefore sensitivity. Thus, appropriate stimuli such as thermal, tactile or osmotic stimuli induce a rapid and marked increase in fluid flow in dentinal tubules. This flow induces a mechanoreceptor response in the A-delta pulpal nerve fibres and pain is perceived. Therefore for this mechanism to operate tubules must be open at the surface and patent to the pulp.

The diameter of the tubules is the major variable controlling flow since, according to Poisseuille's Law, fluid flow is dependent on the fourth power of the tubule radius, i.e. a tubule whose diameter is twice that of another will permit, under the same stimulus, 16 times the fluid flow.

Desensitising toothpastes could contain ingredients which:

- Directly block the tubules.
- Indirectly block tubules by precipitating natural substances in the tubules, e.g. proteins or calcium salts.
- Abrade dentine to form a smear layer.
- Stimulate secondary dentine formation.
- Block pulpal nerve activity.

**40** Listerine contains a mixture of the following compounds: thymol (0·06%), eucalyptol (0·09%), methyl salicyclate (0·06%), and methanol (0·04%) in 26·9% alcohol. Thymol and eucalyptol are phenolic compounds, whereas methyl salicyclate is anti-inflammatory.

The phenolic compounds exert a non-specific antibacterial action which is dependent upon their ability, in the non-ionised form, to penetrate the lipid component of the bacterial cell wall. The resultant structural damage will affect the permeability control of micro-organisms. In addition, several metabolic processes that are dependent upon enzymes contained within the cell membrane, will be inactivated. Phenolic compounds, together with methyl salicyclate have also been shown to exhibit anti-inflammatory properties. These may result from their ability to inhibit neutrophil chemotaxis, the generation of superoxide anions and the production of prostaglandin synthetase. Listerine is particularly useful in long-term chronic gingival conditions. Its antibacterial action is more pronounced against Gram-negative micro-organisms.

**41** In the unfortunate event of a needlestick injury the wound should be held under running water and allowed to bleed. A 10ml sample of blood should be taken from the patient, if known and if consent given, and sent to the local virus laboratory to be tested for Hepatitis B antigen titre. 10ml should also be taken from the DSA and sent to be tested for Hepatitis B antibody. Help should be obtainable by telephoning the Occupational Health Department of the local hospital.

Most needlestick injuries happen to young and inexperienced personnel. It is important in the first instance to prevent them by establishing safe working procedures and to ensure that these are observed throughout the practice. For example, after use, needles should either be re-sheathed using one of the proprietary devices, placed on a working surface, or removed with a pair of Spencer-Wells forceps and then discarded in the sharps bin. Needles should NEVER be resheathed by holding the syringe in one hand and the sheath in the other. This practice is a very common cause of needlestick injury. Similarly, DSAs should always wear heavy duty rubber gloves when cleaning instruments after use. Better still, dirty instruments should be cleaned in an ultrasonic cleaner before autoclaving.

Accurate records of all such accidents must be recorded in the practice Accident Book.

**42** (a) Gingival lichen planus and associated skin lesions. The buccal mucosa (42B) is typical of lichen planus and demonstrates the 'Wickham's striae' that characterise this condition.
(b) (i) Ortho/parakeratinisation of epithelium. (ii) Acanthosis. (iii) 'Saw toothed' rete pegs. (iv) Basal cell liquefaction degeneration. (v) Civatte bodies, hyalinised degenerate cells within the epithelial layer. (vi) Band-like inflammatory infiltrate of the underlying connective tissue. (vii) Subepithelial oedema and occasionally bullae.

**43** (a) (i) The swelling should be removed completely down to the bone. (ii) Pregnancy epulides are frequently associated with mechanical plaque retention factors such as overhangs or calculus. Great attention should be paid to the removal of these leaving a smooth tooth surface. (iii) The wound should be dressed using a periodontal dressing which exerts some pressure. Coe-Pak with cotton wool incorporated is excellent for this purpose. It may be held in place with a floss-silk ligature if likely to be displaced. (iv) The dressing should be changed weekly until the wound is completely epithelised—usually at 2 weeks. If the dressing is removed prematurely, the area will bleed on tooth cleaning, and the patient is likely not to clean properly, if at all. The epulis may then recur rapidly. (v) When the wound is finally left undressed, the patient should be guided carefully in postoperative care, particularly in interdental cleaning and the use of locally applied chlorhexidine. Initially, recall should be at weekly intervals.
(b) The pregnancy epulis is essentially a pyogenic granuloma. The histological picture is one of many endothelium-lined vascular spaces with proliferation of fibroblasts and endothelial cells. The epithelium is ulcerated with a dense inflammatory cell infiltrate.

**44** (a) She has a high lip line with relatively short, broad front teeth. The location of the gingival margin is not yet in its 'mature' position as she is only 9 years of age. In the normal young adult the gingival margin should be approximately 1 mm coronal to the amelo-cemental junction.
(b) Reassurance—but no active treatment is required at present. Orthodontic treatment may be required subsequently as mild potential crowding is apparent. If, following maturation of the gingival margins at late teenage stage, the patient is still concerned about the appearance, then crown lengthening procedures could be considered.

**45** An alternative local delivery method is irrigation using syringes or irrigating devices.
Advantages of local delivery over systemic methods: (i) Markedly reduced total dosage and therefore the possibility of side-effects peculiar to the agent. (ii) Site specific. (iii) Compliance since the therapy is largely operator- and not patient-controlled. (iv) Possible to employ agents unsuitable for systemic application, e.g. antiseptics. (v) Little possibility of super-infection by organisms resistant to antibacterials, e.g. *Candida*. (vi) Little or no possibility of drug interactions with concomitant pharmacotherapy.

Shared disadvantages of local and systemic antimicrobial therapies: (i) emergence of resistant organisms; (ii) allergic or hypersensitivity reactions; (iii) failure to provide long-term adjunctive benefits to conventional mechanical therapies.

Minocycline and metronidazole are currently available for subgingival placement using disposable syringes.

**46** (a) Preferential dentine loss where this is exposed would suggest an erosive factor, the stepped lesions on the palatal surfaces of the upper anterior teeth are related to functional contact with the lower incisors and showing evidence of surrounding tooth faceting confirms a parafunctional element. The differential diagnosis is between the potential etiology of the tooth erosion superimposed upon the parafunctional bruxing activity. Erosion could be related to gastric reflux activity and in a patient of this age, prompt investigation of the patient's weight, sodium/potassium balance and attitude towards food consumption habits. The erosion could be related to dietary factors, however, and consideration should be given to the consumption of fruit juices, carbonated drinks, fruit (particularly citrus), yoghurt, dry wine, cider- or vinegar-containing sauces and preserved vegetables. Remember chewing vitamin C tablets (ascorbic acid) is not unknown. Finally, the patient's employment should be investigated.

Consideration should be given to oral hygiene activities since acid contact with the teeth followed by toothbrushing will contribute to an increased rate of wear.

(b) (i) The patient should be counselled about erosive dietary components and advised:
● To avoid between-meal consumption.
● To avoid cleaning teeth after meals when acid components have been consumed
● To reduce the quantity of acidic food and drink in the diet.
● To complete any meal when acidic components have been consumed with an alkali material such as cheese or milk to assist the buffering capacity of the saliva.
(ii) Gastric reflux activity should be investigated with the help of the patient's general medical practitioner. Toothbrushing following such activity should be avoided. (iii) Environmental erosive factors should be prevented by the Health and Safety at Work Act, usually necessitating the individual to wear appropriate nose and mouth protection. It should be remembered, however, that many such acidic atmospheres (in the silver plating industry, for example) are hot, and carbonated drinks are often used to quench the thirst. (iv) Since the diagnosis includes an element of parafunctional activity which will take place predominantly while asleep at night, a heat-cured resin occlusal appliance of the Michigan type should be worn at night and wear of the appliance surface should be scrutinised regularly to confirm it is being used. (v) Study casts should be taken, dated and stored for further comparison in order to confirm that the preventive measures that have been taken are effective.

**47** The radio-opaque substance in the alveolar bone is polysulphide rubber which has entered the tissues via a break in the epithelial attachment during impression taking. This happened because the preparation was considerably subgingival and much force had necessarily been used to pack retraction cord into the area to obtain a satisfactory impression of the margin of the cavity.

There was a delay of 2 weeks before the rubber base could be removed because the patient was a student and was taking examinations. A buccal flap was raised to reveal a massive area of bone destruction filled with granulation tissue. The wound subsequently healed well with evidence of good bone regeneration.

The damage is caused by lead sulphide in the impression material. This is a powerful oxidising agent and tissue irritant. In this case the impression material entered the bone via the perforations in the alveolar crest. In other cases on record the material has come to lie as a sheet between the bone and the periosteum on the facial or oral side of the jaw, when it shows up on the radiograph as an oval area of increased radio-opacity.

Problems like this should not occur now. It is generally accepted that the margins of cavities should be supragingival where they are accessible for cleaning by the patient. The only exceptions to this are for reasons of aesthetics in the case of an anterior restoration, for purposes of retention, or where caries, a previous restoration or fracture dictate a subgingival finish.

Damage to the periodontal structures as illustrated in this case has also been recorded following the process of 'troughing', where electrosurgery is used to remove the wall of the gingival crevice adjacent to a cavity margin in order to obtain a good impression of a subgingival cavity margin easily.

**48** His oral hygiene is infrequent and he has a marked tendency towards calculus formation. The reason for the calculus distribution is that he is right-handed with poor manual dexterity. His cleaning of the right side of his mouth is therefore less efficient than the left.

**49** The bone loss mesial to 47 is clearly advanced and there is unlikely to be massive regeneration following conventional periodontal therapy, although guided tissue regeneration may result in significant new attachment. However this is an ideal case for hemisection. The furcation is high, the distal root is long and well supported by bone and the distal root canal is clearly visible and capable of being root-filled after vital extirpation of the pulp.

After root-filling of the distal root, a buccal flap was raised to expose the bifurcation and the tooth sectioned from the bifurcation to the occlusal surface. It is important always to cut from the bifurcation and not towards it—the latter procedure often results in loss of direction and either removal of too much or too little tooth substance. When the two halves are separate—this can be checked by gently twisting a straight Warwick–James elevator in the cut—the mesial root can be extracted with forceps.

The wound was sutured and after healing a fixed–fixed bridge was constructed on the remaining root of 47 and 45.

**50** (a) Grossly widened periodontal ligament space, root resorption and calcification in pulp chamber of 11.
(b) Primary occlusal trauma.
(c) Maintain periodontal health by reinforcing oral hygiene instructions (efficient use of brush, tape and disclosing solution). Occlusal analysis and adjustment to remove any premature contacts. Fit a bite guard for night wear. Splinting of 11 is possible but is unlikely to extend the life of the tooth.

**51** (a) Acute lymphoblastic leukaemia. This is predominantly a disease of childhood with peak incidence from the age of 3 to 5 years. It is the most common childhood malignancy. Some degree of anaemia and thrombocytopenia is always found but the white blood cell (WBC) count is very variable. The WBC count may be decreased, normal or increased, but leukaemic blast cells are always seen in the blood smear. High WBC counts indicate a poorer prognosis. There are often marked gingival changes in acute myeloblastic anaemia with gingival swelling and leukaemic cell infiltration. This is less common in the lymphoblastic type where pallor of the mucosa is usually seen.
(b) The goal of treatment is to achieve complete remission. The regimes involved are complex and ideally patients should be treated at specialised centres. Cytotoxic drugs, including vincristine, L-asparaginase, cyclophosphamide, doxorubicin and methotrexate are given with daily prednisolone. An important site of leukaemic infiltration is the meninges and treatment may, therefore, include intrathecal methotrexate plus cranial irradiation. Supportive treatment includes blood transfusions, etc., and a bone marrow transplant may be required in cases of relapse.

(c) Oral care is designed to minimise and palliate the side-effects of the systemic treatment. If dental treatment is required in the acute phase of the disease, it should be limited to emergency care until the patient is in remission. A very high standard of oral hygiene is necessary to minimise the oral ulceration which tends to arise from the chemotherapy. Unfortunately the children always feel nauseous at this stage of the treatment and oral cleansing is difficult. Chlorhexidine spray and swabs are helpful along with benzydamine hydrochloride spray. Antifungal agents are prescribed routinely.

**52** (a) This is an amalgam tattoo.
(b) It arises when silver amalgam is inadvertently introduced into the gingival tissues, then phagocytosed, and the silver stains released into the tissues.
(c) A radiograph to confirm that there is no underlying pathology.
(d) Reassurance that the lesion is benign and only a cosmetic blemish.

**53** The gingival enlargement is a pregnancy epulis; the unfortunate alternative term 'pregnancy tumour' should not be used. The more generalised gingival condition is pregnancy gingivitis. Pregnancy itself does not cause these conditions but merely modifies the response of the gingivae to the aetiological factor, namely bacterial plaque. The hormonal changes appear to enhance the inflammatory response of the gingivae to plaque such that increased redness and swelling occur. Usually therefore gingivitis pre-exists in these women. Post-partum both pregnancy epulides and gingivitis show marked and spontaneous regression. For this reason management should be where possible conservative in nature. Oral hygiene advice and simple local debridement is all that is indicated. If frank deposits of supra- or subgingival calculus are present these should be removed. However, it is surprising how little resolution occurs until post-partum. Removal of epulides should be avoided unless they are so large as to interfere with function and/or the occlusion or are a major aesthetic problem. If removal is necessary before parturition, bleeding is usually quite profuse and cautery or lasers may be the method of choice.

**54** (i) Although pregnancy epulides generally regress after pregnancy, they rarely regress completely.
(ii) If removed completely and proper steps are taken to prevent recurrence, they rarely return.
(iii) Good local anaesthesia with adequate vasoconstriction prevents excessive bleeding during removal.
(iv) They can be very unsightly.
(v) They may interfere with function and bleed when the patient is eating.
(vi) They may continue to grow very rapidly, as in this case.
(vii) The lesion may not be a pregnancy epulis but something more sinister (e.g. an osteogenic sarcoma or other malignant tumour). Surgical removal allows the epulis to be examined histologically.

**55** Diagnosis: prepubertal periodontitis.
Clinical findings:
(i) Inflammatory signs:
● Intense red appearance of gingivae.
● Marginal and attached gingivae affected.
● Gingival cleft formation and recession.
(ii) Rapid alveolar bone destruction with resultant premature loss of primary dentition.

(iii) Haematologically:
- Increased peripheral WBC count.
- Functional defects of peripheral blood neutrophils and/or monocytes.

**56** (a) Eruption cyst.
(b) Most of these lesions should more accurately be called eruption haematomas as they consist of blood extravasated into the soft tissues overlying a newly erupting tooth and are not lined by epithelium—the true definition of a cyst. They usually appear to be bluish in colour, dome-shaped and fluctuant. However, the one shown here could be considered as a minor soft tissue form of a follicular cyst. It is fluctuant and has arisen from separation of the dental follicle from around the anatomical crown of the unerupted tooth.
(c) No treatment is usually required as they normally burst spontaneously. The 'old-fashioned' remedies of hard teething toys and hard sugar-free rusks are useful in young children. Hard, fibrous foods encouraged the discharge of this one and eruption of the left central incisor then proceeded normally. Very rarely they may become symptomatic or appear to be delaying eruption, in these cases excision of an ellipse of overlying gingiva may be required.

**57** Air polishers work by directing particles of sodium bicarbonate contained in a jet of air and water onto the tooth surface. They are very effective indeed in removing a stubborn extrinsic stain such as that produced by tobacco or chlorhexidine mouthwash.
   They do, however, abrade the gingival tissues, causing bleeding and damage exposed root surface. If used with only a saliva ejector for moisture control purposes they create considerable atmospheric pollution. Rinsing with a chlorhexidine mouthwash for 2 minutes before the machine is used reduces the atmospheric microbial count by two-thirds. Pollution control is best achieved, however, by use of high volume suction which can reduce the microbial count almost to resting levels.

**58** The instruments are plastic scalers and are used for removing calculus from implants. It is most important that the titanium implant is kept calculus-free by regular scaling but it must not be scratched. They are made of heat-resistant plastic which is not damaged by autoclaving.

**59** The instrument is usually referred to as a WHO probe but was originally called a CPITN probe, intended for recording the Community Periodontal Index of Treatment Needs. It is now widely used for carrying out the basic periodontal examination (BPE). This examination assesses the presence or absence of gingival bleeding, calculus or overhangs and pathologic pockets. The probe is used with a force of 20–25g.
   The probe's special features are:
(i) A ball end 0·5mm in diameter which reduces the risk of penetrating the base of the pocket as may happen with a sharp probe.
(ii) A coloured band between 3·5mm and 5·5mm from the ball end.
(iii) This version of the probe (intended for clinical rather than epidemiological purposes) has a second coloured band between 8·5 and 11·5mm.

**60** In this instance, the root was removed because the tooth had been root-filled some years previously and subsequently developed an apical abscess on the disto-buccal root, which presented as a combined periodontal endodontic lesion with pocketing to the apex.
   Other reasons for root resection in the case of an upper molar are very deep pocketing affecting only one root, bone loss in the furcation where removal of one root may be reasonably expected to produce a cleanable tooth contour postoperatively or where

endodontic treatment proves impossible in the case of one root.

Careful diagnosis and treatment planning are necessary when contemplating root resection. It is necessary to ensure that the roots are completely separate and that those to be left are adequately root-filled.

**61** The reason for the different rates of plaque regrowth is that the upper subject has perfectly healthy periodontal tissues while the lower one has pre-existing gingivitis. In the latter case the quantity of gingival crevicular fluid produced is considerably increased resulting in the presence at the gingival margin of an ideal culture medium for bacterial growth. The clinical implication is that in all patients with periodontal disease of any degree of severity, plaque will reform rapidly after removal and therefore patients should be instructed to carry out thorough plaque control twice daily.

**62** The lesion is an acute *herpes simplex* infection of the finger. The photograph was taken before clinicians routinely wore gloves during treatment of patients, and the dentist concerned had recently treated a patient with a recurrent cold sore, or *herpes labialis*. This case highlights the importance of wearing gloves during clinical work to avoid infection of the operator. Gloves also prevent infection of the patient via minute cuts on the operator's hand. Changing gloves between patients eliminates the risk of infection being transferred from one patient to another via the hands of the clinician. In cases of such infection, clinical work should not be undertaken until the lesion has healed.

**63** The abnormalities are dehiscence (in association with 33) and fenestration (in association with 34). Both are developmental in origin and occur when teeth erupt labially, or more rarely, lingually in the arch, or as in this case, where the investing bone is slender. The significance of dehiscence is that it predisposes to gingival recession. When the tooth erupts, the overlying gingival tissue will be normal, but damage arising as a result of over-vigorous toothbrushing or plaque-induced gingivitis will result in the junctional or pocket epithelium fusing with the external gingival epithelium resulting in a vertical slit, known in the past as a Stillman's cleft. This then proceeds to gingival recession which will continue until the bone margin is reached when the gingival margin stabilises, albeit at a more apical level.

Fenestration, which is a circumscribed area of missing bone, is of little significance except when bone loss is advancing and encounters such an area when a pocket may be expected to deepen suddenly.

It is possible that dehiscence and fenestration could be caused by faulty orthodontic treatment but in practice this is probably uncommon.

**64** (a) Direct structural and functional connection between ordered, living bone and the surface of a load-bearing implant.
(b) Titanium oxide present on the surface of commercially pure titanium. Some would also claim that osseointegration also occurs with hydroxyapatite used to coat some titanium implants. Although this may be true in the short term, after a period of time the hydroxy-apatite is broken down and resorbed.
(c) Because of the danger of scratching and roughening the implant abutment, plastic instruments are recommended. The calculus is not difficult to remove.
(d) An improvement in oral hygiene. The superstructure should be designed to give easy access for cleaning. A small soft toothbrush should be used for most of the cleaning. An interdental or bottle-type brush of a suitable size can be used to clean under and around the abutments. If calculus formation is a problem, an 'anti-tartar' toothpaste containing diphosphonates could be recommended.

65  The incidence and severity of postoperative pain after periodontal surgery, when compared with other dental surgical procedures, is low. Most patients experience pain in the early postoperative period (i.e. when the effects of the local anaesthetic have worn off). After 24 hours, the pain experience is usually minimal. The surgical procedure induces a localised inflammatory response resulting in the release of the eicosanoids (especially prostaglandins and the leukotrienes), histamine and bradykinin. Pain production arises as a result of an interaction between prostaglandins of the E series, histamine and bradykinin. Prostaglandins sensitise the free nerve endings to the nociceptive properties of histamine and bradykinin. This results in pain at or near the site of injury.

The inflammatory nature of postoperative pain after periodontal surgery indicates that drugs with an analgesic and anti-inflammatory action are the treatment of choice. In addition, the anti-inflammatory properties will help to reduce local swelling which often accompanies such surgery. Aspirin (600–1200mg) or ibuprofen (400mg) are efficacious, and soluble preparations provide a more rapid onset of analgesia. For patients who cannot take aspirin or ibuprofen (i.e. asthmatics or patients with a history of peptic ulceration), paracetamol is a useful alternative. The latter drug lacks the anti-inflammatory properties of either aspirin or ibuprofen.

66  (a) Chlorhexidine is inhibitory to a wide range of oral micro-organisms, including Gram-positive and Gram-negative bacteria, and yeasts (such as *Candida* species).
(b) Chlorhexidine is particularly active against *Streptococcus mutans*, one of the bacteria associated with dental caries.
(c) Chlorhexidine at high concentrations has a bactericidal effect and acts as a detergent by damaging the cell membrane, leading to precipitation of cytoplasmic contents. At lower concentrations, it may have other effects on oral bacteria, including inhibition of sugar intake and modification of metabolic activity.
(d) Chlorhexidine binds to teeth, dental plaque bacteria and other surfaces in the oral cavity, from which it may exert prolonged bacteriostatic activity. This phenomenon of adsorption followed by slow release, resulting in persistence of antimicrobial effects, is sometimes referred to as 'substantivity'.
(e) Some people find the bitter taste of chlorhexidine unpleasant, and oral preparations tend to cause staining of the teeth. Long-term suppression of the normal oral flora by chlorhexidine or any other antimicrobial agent carries a risk of overgrowth or colonisation by 'undesirable' micro-organisms, and the emergence of potentially dangerous resistant strains. As a general rule, the use of such antimicrobial agents should be reserved for specific clinical situations and courses of treatment should not be prolonged indefinitely.

67  The instruments are calculus probes. The lower one is a Cross probe, the upper a Hu–Friedy. The WHO probe with its ball end tends to slide over small deposits of calculus and is not as good at detecting surface roughness after root planing as specifically designed calculus detection probes. The Hu–Friedy probe is especially valuable for use in areas which are difficult to access such as furcations. These probes can also detect other root surface abnormalities such as developmental grooves.

68  Green stain is occasionally seen on the teeth of children with poor oral hygiene—it is believed to be caused by chromogenic bacteria. Stain in adults is usually brown or black and is caused by tobacco-smoking, drinking of tea, coffee or red wine and the use of mouthwashes containing chlorhexidine.

In this case, the patient is a maker and polisher of brass ornaments and the green colour is caused by the inclusion of copper salts into the pellicle.

**69** (a) (i) Full clinical examination including pocket depth measurements. (ii) Radiographs: periapical radiographs in the incisor region combined with an orthopantomogram initially. (iv) Full mouth periapicals may be required. (v) Haematological screening, immunological investigation, urine analysis and biopsy.

(b) Intense oral hygiene instruction, with root planing and use of chlorhexidine in the first instance. The further treatment depends on the response to this initial care and on the results from the haematological screening, etc. In this particular patient there was an initial improvement but a further deterioration after 2 weeks. Tetracycline was then prescribed, although its use in this situation is controversial and it should never be used in children under the age of about 7 years because of the risk of staining. The response to this was disappointing and finally a biopsy and thorough root planing were carried out under a general anaesthetic.

(c) Pre-pubertal periodontitis. This may occur in conjunction with juvenile-onset diabetes, hyperparathyroidism, adrenocortical hyperfunction (Cushing's syndrome), scleroderma, histiocytosis X and Papillon-Lefèvre syndrome.

N.B. Nothing in the initial clinical, radiological or haematological investigations suggested that this pre-pubertal periodontitis was associated with any of these conditions. However, the lack of response to the initial treatment should raise the 'clinical index of suspicion'. The biopsy showed a dense infiltrate of inflammatory cells, the majority of which were histiocytes, hence a diagnosis of histiocytosis X of the gingiva was made and the patient referred to a consultant paediatric oncologist.

**70** The brush is an interdental brush for cleaning interdentally. For patients who have periodontitis with loss of interdental bone and resultant recession, it is probably the easiest method of interdental cleaning. The bristles enter the gingival crevice and will clean for a short distance subgingivally. The other methods of cleaning interdentally are the use of floss or tape. Their use needs to be taught to the patient carefully since improper use can be damaging or ineffectual. Many patients never master the art of using floss or tape properly and where this is the case, use of the interdental brush is a good alternative where possible. Floss and tape are obtainable in waxed and unwaxed forms. Waxed forms are easier to use since the unwaxed varieties tend to shred when used on teeth with restorations which have imperfect margins.

**71** The patient 'did not believe in' using toothpaste and instead brushed his teeth using toilet soap. This case illustrates the need for the inclusion of a polishing agent in dentifrices to remove or prevent the build-up of pellicle, which in this case has developed into a thick layer and become stained by constituents of the diet, except for 11 which is a porcelain jacket crown. Pellicle does not form on glazed porcelain.

**72** (i) Periapical cemental dysplasia. (ii) Gigantiform cementoma. (iii) Benign cementoblastoma. (iv) Cementifying fibroma.

Of these, periapical cemental dysplasia is the most likely. It is most common in black females over the age of 20 and usually occurs in and around the periodontal ligament at the apex of mandibular incisor teeth and is often multiple. At its earliest stage the lesion forms a periapical radiolucency, where bone is lost and replaced with fibrous tissue, the so-called 'osteolytic phase'. Usually teeth are vital and no treatment is indicated. In this case the periodontic/endodontic lesion is probably coincidental. The second or 'cementoblastic phase' involves calcification within the radiolucent lesion leading to a mixed radiolucent/radio-opaque appearance. The third or 'mature phase' involves excessive calcification and a definite radiopaque appearance. No treatment is indicated, unless there is another lesion involved. This tooth was extracted, but the cementoma remained behind and was left in place.

**73** This is a giant cell epulis or peripheral giant cell granuloma. Given the history and, at first observation, the appearance of the lesion, a pregnancy epulis would be a reasonable diagnosis. However, the colour of the lesion is more purple than red and some history of bleeding would be expected. More importantly, there is evidence of displacement of the teeth to either side of the lesion and this would be most unusual for an inflammatory epulis. The most likely alternative diagnosis given the appearance and history would be a giant cell epulis. With either diagnosis a possibility at this stage of the pregnancy, a delay in treatment until post-partum is indicated. The lack of any resolution in the lesion post-partum would not be consistent with a pregnancy epulis. A radiograph can now be safely requested and this revealed considerable bone loss between the lateral incisor and canine, a feature sometimes observed with peripheral giant cell lesions*. The lesion should be excised and the bony base thoroughly curetted. There was no recurrence on follow-up.
* Haematological tests for serum calcium and phosphate in combination with serum alkaline phosphatase levels would exclude hyperparathyroidism as a cause.

**74** The protuberance is apparently composed of enamel (an enameloma) and is acting as a retention factor for subgingival plaque. It was decided to remove it with a diamond bur to leave a smooth dentine surface for reattachment to occur. This was accomplished successfully at first but the tooth subsequently developed an apical abscess. This must have been due to a prolongation of pulp into the lesion which was checked for at operation but not seen. Following root-filling, the tooth has remained symptomless. Such dental 'lumps' should always be checked carefully for pulpal extensions.

**75** Prescribing to the breast-feeding mother can result in the drug passing from the maternal circulation, through the mammary gland epithelium and into the breast milk. Thus the baby will be exposed to the maternal drug, which may cause unwanted effects in the child. Drugs in breast milk can have the following effects:
(i) an adverse effect on the baby; (ii) inhibition of the sucking reflex; (iii) alteration of the taste of the milk; (iv) the development of drug hypersensitivity.
   In dentistry, the following drugs should be avoided:
   *Aspirin*—high doses of aspirin enter the breast milk and can cause impairment of platelet aggregation in the baby.
   *Tetracycline*—prolonged usage, as may occur in the management of certain types of periodontal disease, can cause intrinsic staining of the teeth, impaired bone growth and alteration of the gut flora.
   *Penicillins*—can provoke a hypersensitivity reaction in a previously sensitised baby. Ampicillin taken by nursing mothers, can cause diarrhoea and candidiasis in the breast-fed child.
   *Metronidazole*—can give breast milk a bitter taste.

**76** (a) The periodontitis on the upper right central incisor (11) has progressed and now involves the apex of the tooth. This is now a potential or actual periodontic/endodontic lesion.
(b) The pocket depths should be charted and related to the radiographic detail. A pulp test should also be undertaken to assess the vitality of the tooth.
(c) This lesion is too deep to be accessible for root planing. A periodontal flap will be required to enable root surface debridement. This would undoubtedly lead to loss of vitality of the pulp, so if this type of treatment is contemplated, then root canal therapy should be undertaken first. The prognosis for the tooth must be guarded.

(d) Initially a provisional immediate plastic denture. The adventurous could consider removing the root of the tooth and retrograde filling the remaining crown, which would be retained in the splint. In the long run the decision would be between a spoon denture, a metal-based denture or a fixed restoration, most appropriately of the acid-etch retained type.

**77** (a) White sponge naevus (oral epithelial naevus). This condition is hereditary and may be present in infancy or later in childhood. It can affect any part of the oral mucosa and the creamy ragged lesions vary in thickness. Histologically, there is marked parakeratosis and this builds up to produce the clinically roughened, keratotic appearance. The epithelium is acanthotic, there is intracellular oedema and generally no inflammation of the lamina propria.
(b) No treatment is indicated and there is no evidence for malignant transformation.

**78** There is furcation involvement of the first molar. Furcation involvements of upper molar and first premolar teeth are more easily missed on radiographs than those affecting lower molar teeth, because of superimposition. They are also of greater significance in their effect on treatment and prognosis. Whether suspected or not, a search for furcation involvements should be a feature of all periodontal assessments. This involves probing all potentially affected areas, not forgetting the lingual aspects of lower molars. They are graded 1, 2 or 3 according to whether a probe will just enter the furcation area (1), enter to a depth greater than 2mm horizontally (2), or pass all the way through the furcation (3).

**79** Diagnosis: acute necrotising ulcerative periodontitis.
Clinical features:
- Bleeding gums.
- Foul taste.
- Loosening of teeth.
- Rapid regression often within a few weeks.
- This condition is usually very painful.
- Soft tissue loss due to ulceration and necrosis.
- Bone may be exposed in defects and consequently be sequestered.
- Tissue destruction may extend beyond mucogingival junction.
- May not respond to routine periodontal treatment.

**80** (a) Cyclic (periodic) neutropenia. In this condition the level of circulating neutrophils is relatively normal for periods of 3 weeks, but then falls for 5–8 days. In this latter period, recurrent infections occur. These characteristically involve the oral mucosa, the periodontium, the upper respiratory tract and the urogenital tract.
In general, neutropenias may be persistent, cyclic or transient. The majority of neutropenias are due to abnormalities in the bone marrow, and can result from direct injury or from maturational defects in haemopoietic cells. Chemical injury is common from substances such as benzene, dinitrophenol and DDT. Maturational defects may be primary (hereditary) or secondary (e.g. folic or vitamin $B_{12}$ deficiency).
(b) Differential white blood cells counts at weekly intervals for at least 4 weeks.
(c) Periodontal treatment of patients with cyclic neutropenia demands meticulous attention to detail. Thorough scaling should be carried out and the patient should be encouraged to carry out plaque control to a high standard. In addition to brushing the patient should use dental floss or tape, and chlorhexidine mouthwashes will help with supragingival plaque control. If after such treatment any bleeding sites remain, root planing should be carried

out. Treatment of refractory problems may require systemic antibiotic therapy (e.g. with co-amoxycyclav), but this should always be done in conjunction with the patient's physician. The patient should be seen at 3-monthly intervals for maintenance; long-term maintenance may be aided by the use of an irrigating device with a 50:50 solution of chlorhexidine 0·2% and water.

81 (a) Ehlers–Danlos syndrome.
(b) This has an autosomal dominant inheritance.
(c) (i) Short, tapering, fragile roots. These predispose the teeth to fracture when extracted.
(ii) Susceptible to periodontal disease because of the inherited connective tissue defect. (iii) Post-tooth extraction haemorrhage. (iv) Early obliteration of the pulp chambers with loss of pulp vitality and apical abscess formation.

82 The primary aim for successful treatment of chronic periodontal disease is thorough debridement of the root surface to remove subgingival plaque deposits. Surgical treatment merely acts to permit the root surface to be observed and therefore can facilitate the debridement procedure. Most if not all studies indicate that closed root planing is as effective as surgery with root planing and particularly effective when single rooted teeth are involved. Additionally, loss of attachment is less with non-surgical techniques compared to surgical methods. In the case presented here, this could be of aesthetic importance in the upper anterior region where surgically induced recession may compromise appearance. Root planing, however, may be difficult to perform effectively around multi-rooted teeth, particularly with furcation involvement or where the pattern of bone loss renders it difficult or impossible to instrument to the apical limit of the lesion.

83 (a) Root canal treatment of the remaining teeth, crown reductions and dome preparations and, of course, provision of an overdenture.
(b) Cleaning of the roots and gingivae with a soft brush using a fluoride-containing toothpaste. If caries is a problem, the patient could be shown how to apply a fluoride gel to the root surfaces. The tongue has a coating so advice on cleaning the anterior area of the dorsum would also be appropriate.
(c) It should be removed for cleaning at least twice a day, morning and night. A soft toothbrush with a non-scented soap could be used for cleaning. If staining occurs, then a hypochlorite-containing denture cleaner could be used overnight. Unless there are other problems, such as temporomandibular joint (TMJ) dysfunction or myofacial pain, the denture should be left out at night, but kept moist.
(d) Improved support and stability. Reduced alveolar ridge resorption, which increases the interval between relines or remakes. There is a considerable psychological benefit from retaining teeth, as well as improved proprioception.

84 Modern concepts of periodontal disease and its progression are as follows:
(i) Most gingivitis remains contained for many years. It has never been shown that gingivitis always proceeds to periodontitis, nor has it been shown that periodontitis is invariably preceded by gingivitis.
(ii) Severe destructive periodontitis affects only a relatively small proportion of the population. Suggestions are that this is approximately 10–12%.
(iii) The disease is highly site-specific. It is not uncommon to find terminal bone loss affecting one or more teeth in a mouth while others exhibit perfect periodontal health. Equally, one surface of a tooth may exhibit advanced disease while another surface is unaffected.

(iv) Most periodontitis is in long-term remission.

(v) Progression of periodontitis is believed to be episodic with periods of activity, inactivity and even healing following each other.

**85** (a) Good history of the pain and swelling. Extra-oral examination for swelling, bony inconsistencies, evidence of trauma. Intra-oral examination: check the nature and extent of the pain and swelling and the presence of any discharge. Swab any discharge to identify causative organisms. Check plaque control, periodontal indices and pocketing around implants. Check for any trauma or food impaction. Check for mobility of the bridge or abutments and the occlusion. Radiographic investigation to screen for incomplete seating of implant abutment, fractured bone or implant components and excessive loss of crestal bone.

(b) Peri-implantitis.

(c) Poor oral hygiene leading to the development of a 'periodontopathic' subgingival flora.Trauma from toothbrushing or food impaction, especially where the implant is encompassed by mobile alveolar mucosa and the gingival cuff is deep. Incomplete seating of the implant abutment allows plaque to collect and be retained in an inaccessible subgingival site. Similarly, fracture of fixture of abutment components will cause mechanical and bacteriological irritation of the implant cuff.

(d) Depending upon the extent of the swelling and pain, and provided any implant/abutment inconsistencies have been corrected, the peri-implantitis can often be managed by local means alone, such as scaling, pocket irrigation and an appropriate standard of plaque control. In cases of severe swelling and discomfort, or where there is evidence of continuing alveolar crestal loss, then systemic antimicrobial therapy (e.g. oxytetracycline, metronidazole or amoxycillin) is appropriate.

**86** This is a case of Wegener's granulomatosis presenting as a hyperplastic 'strawberry' gingivitis. Biopsy is essential in such cases. A further diagnostic feature in Wegener's granulomatosis is the presence of anticytoplasmic antibodies to the intracytoplasmic antigens of neutrophils. This forms the basis of the ANCA test. The ESR is also raised in these cases.

Systemic involvement of Wegener's granulomatosis can be life-threatening. Lesions include necrotising granulomas in the nose, paranasal sinuses and lungs, vasculitis of small arteries and veins, and glomerulitis characterised by necrosis of loops of the glomerular tufts, capsular adhesions and granulomatous lesions. The clinical features which can accompany these pathological changes include an intractable rhinitis and sinusitis, cough, haemoptysis and terminal uraemia. Thus such patients should be referred to a physician for renal and pulmonary screening. The disease responds to immunosuppressive therapy of prednisolone and cyclophosphamide.

**87** Data from epidemiological studies suggests that patients who smoke exhibit poorer oral hygiene and higher plaque and calculus scores. As a consequence, smokers have more periodontal destruction than age/sex-matched non-smokers. By contrast, cigarette smoking causes reduced gingival bleeding and crevicular fluid flow. This is attributable to the actions of nicotine on the muscarinic receptors on blood vessels. Activation of these receptors causes vasoconstriction.

Smoking increases the anaerobic environment in the mouth and thus an increased occurrence of acute necrotising ulcerative gingivitis. There is also evidence to suggest that smoking causes delayed wound healing and impaired white blood cell chemotaxis.

**88** (a) Loss of tooth substance may occur by one of the following mechanisms, or by a combination of any two, or by all three: attrition, abrasion, erosion.
(b) In investigating attrition the patient should be questioned about any parafunctional habits. Extra-oral examination should assess any hypertrophy of the facial muscles and the presence of temporomandibular joint symptoms such as pain, noise or altered function. Intra-oral examination should assess the extent and amount of loss of tooth substance, basic periodontal examination (BPE), mobility and migration of teeth, and evidence of cheek or tongue biting. In addition, abrasion requires investigation of oral hygiene methods and materials used, and erosion requires questioning about any gastrointestinal symptoms, charting of any cavities and dietary investigation.

**89** (a) Acute atrophic candidiasis.
(b) The effect of topical steroids upon the oral mucosa is reported to cause this. This patient used a steroid inhaler for his asthma and the pathway of drug passage maps out the candidal infection.
(c) The patient should rinse his mouth with water thoroughly after inhaler use. Topical or systemic antifungals may be used to treat the presenting infection.
(d) Candidal infections are common as opportunist infections in immunocompromised patients. An underlying immune deficiency should be considered, e.g. HIV infection.

**90** This young lady has a Class II division I malocclusion with a grossly increased overjet. Her lower lip is usually tucked behind the maxillary incisors and she cannot achieve a lip seal. She habitually mouth-breathes. Resultant potential problems include:
(i) Increased overbite may result in a traumatic occlusion of the lower incisors with the palatal mucosa. (ii) The inability to achieve a lip seal results in the drying of the mucosa, particularly in the upper incisor region. This will affect the local host response in the gingiva to the colonisation of bacteria on the tooth surface as gingival exudate and salivary flow are both reduced.

It has been shown that clinically and statistically there is a high and significant increase in the incidence of trauma to upper anterior teeth with increasing overjet.

**91** A simple attack of syncope (faint) is the most likely cause of the patient's symptoms. Obviously, stop administering the local anaesthetic and check that the solution has not been injected into a vein. The patient should be laid flat and the pulse monitored. Get help and watch the airway. If the diagnosis is syncope, then these measures will suffice and the patient will start to feel normal within a few seconds. A glucose drink can then be given and, provided the patient is fully recovered, treatment can be continued.

Syncope due to the administration of a local anaesthetic can be prevented by ensuring that the patient has eaten prior to treatment. The injection is given with the patient in the supine position and an aspirating technique is always carried out.

If the patient does not recover, he has not fainted and the differential diagnosis is either a hypoglycaemic attack or an anaphylactic reaction to the local anaesthetic solution. Hypoglycaemia is treated with intramuscular glucagon and intravenous glucose solution. An acute anaphylactic reaction requires immediate treatment with 0·5ml of 1:1,000 adrenaline given intramuscularly and intravenous hydrocortisone hemisuccinate 100mg.

**92** The lesion is a recurrent cold sore, or herpes labialis. The appearance of the vesicle is preceded for a few hours by an intense localised itching. If the area is treated by applying 5% acyclovir cream every 4 hours the condition can be aborted. While the lesion is present it must be assumed that the virus is replicating and infected squames are being shed. Clinicians therefore must wear a mask at all times if they have a cold sore and are treating patients and must carefully observe precautions to avoid cross-infection. Since herpetic infections can be life-threatening in the case of patients who are immunocompromised, clinical staff should not treat such patients until the cold-sore has healed.

93 (a) Code 3: heavy accumulations of plaque filling the niche between the gingival margin and the tooth surface. The interdental area is filled with debris.
(b) Code 1: plaque present.
(c) Code 1: soft debris covering not more than one-third of the tooth surface.
(d) Score 3: stained debris present in the mesial, distal and bucco-cervical areas.

94 (a) No, HIV-G appears to respond less well to conventional plaque control measures than gingivitis in HIV negative subjects.
(b) Some studies have indicated that the microflora associated with HIV-G is similar to that found in HIV-P, and strikingly different to that found in conventional gingivitis.
(c) Yes, it has been suggested that lesions found in HIV-G may progress rapidly to produce HIV-P and the fact that there are similar, increased levels of known periodontopathic organisms in such lesions supports this view.
(d) The clinical presentation of HIV-P has a number of similarities to ANUG and both conditions are often associated with pain (although the described location of the pain may be different). However, the rapidly progressive course of HIV-P is one distinguishing feature. There is insufficient detailed information available at present to draw firm conclusions about the similarity or otherwise between the microflora associated with HIV-P and ANUG.
(e) Some studies have demonstrated the presence of increased levels of *Porphyromonas gingivalis* (formerly called *Bacteroides gingivalis*), *Prevotella intermedia* (formerly *Bacteroides intermedius*), *Fusobacterium nucleatum*, and *Actinobacillus actinomycetemcomitans* in both HIV-G and HIV-P, compared to normal controls. However, further work is required to clarify the microbial aetiology of these HIV-associated periodontal conditions.

95 (a) The causative agent of chicken pox is the varicella–zoster virus (VZV). It is one of the herpes viruses, which is a large and clinically important group of DNA viruses.
(b) Chicken pox or varicella typically produces a centripetal rash, involving the trunk and the head. The appearance of the rash changes with time, going through macular, papular, vesicular and pustular stages. The average incubation period is 14–15 days (range: 10–20 days) and the patient is infectious from about 2 days before until 5 days after the rash appears.Oral manisfestations may appear at an early stage, before the typical skin rash develops.
(c) A number of viral infections, including some of the other childhood fevers, may produce oral lesions. These include measles, mumps, infectious mononucleosis (Epstein–Barr virus), and Coxsackie A virus infections.
(d) VZV causes shingles (zoster) in some adults.

96 (a) Hairy leukoplakia.
(b) The Epstein–Barr virus has been implicated in the aetiology of hairy leukoplakia. The role of papillomavirus has yet to be confirmed. The lesion may regress when the patient is prescribed a course of acyclovir.

(c) As a clinical manifestation of HIV infection the patient's classification of their condition changes from CDC II (asymptomatic) to CDC III (exhibiting evidence of HIV infection).

(d) Other conditions that mimic the clinical presentation: (i) tobacco-related keratosis; (ii) frictional keratosis; (iii) lichen planus; (iv) idiopathic leukoplakia; (v) candidal leukoplakia; (vi) galvanic lesions

**97** This is a hypersensitivity reaction—the so-called plasma cell gingivitis which is usually caused by spicy foods, toothpastes or chewing gum. It is important to elicit from the patient any recent change in eating habits or toothpaste usage. Biopsy is useful in confirming the diagnosis. The main histopathological finding is a heavy infiltration of plasma cells into the submucosa. Immunofluorescent studies show that most of the mononuclear cells have an antibody halo on the cell membrane surface. These findings, together with the clinical history of sudden onset, confirm the diagnosis.

The condition is usually self-limiting once the suspected allergen has been identified and patch testing may be useful. Patients should be told to discontinue their current toothpaste. Topical corticosteroid may facilitate resolution of the inflammation.

**98** (a) (i) Haemangioma. (ii) Kaposi's sarcoma. (iii) Pyogenic granuloma. (iv) Peripheral/central giant cell granuloma. (v) Erythroplakia. The lesion was, in fact, Kaposi's sarcoma.
(b) If the patient presented in general practice, he should be referred to the nearest hospital for an opinion. An incisional biopsy should be performed, where the diagnosis is clearly unknown and malignancy is suspected. If the lesion is excised wholly and the histopathology is of malignancy, it is difficult to know where the lesion margin was to enable wider excision.
(c) The implications of the histopathology should be explained carefully to the patient who should he be questioned about possible HIV status, homosexuality or intravenous drug abuse, since Kaposi's sarcoma is more common in homosexual AIDS patients. A full medical examination should be arranged together with counselling and HIV testing in the appropriate hospital department. Treatment of oral Kaposi's sarcoma in an HIV-positive patient depends upon the presence or absence of other Kaposi's lesions. If isolated, intralesional chemotherapy can be used (e.g. vinblastine 0·2mg/ml in 0·1ml aliquots per 0·5cm of lesion). Radiotherapy may be used or excision (with extraction of the adjacent teeth). Recently results with a $CO_2$ laser have been impressive. This lesion was treated by radiotherapy and is shown 3 months post-treatment (**98B**). There is residual pigmentation and loss of the labial bone plate as a result of the tumour. The patient's oral health was maintained with regular cleaning and oral hygiene instruction (OHI), including the use of chlorhexidine mouthwash until he died 18 months after initial diagnosis of the gingival Kaposi's lesion. Towards the end of his life the patient found rinsing with the chlorhexidine mouthwash difficult and uncomfortable. Instead his mouth was swabbed with dilute mouthwash.

**99** The patient has been using triangular interdental wood sticks for the last 30 years and these have abraded the interproximal surfaces of the roots exposed as a result of gingival recession secondary to periodontitis. The use of wood sticks was once encouraged as a means of forming a thicker layer of keratin on the interdental papilla. It is now realised that this is irrelevant in the context of the prevention and treatment of periodontal disease. What is important is the removal of plaque, particularly subgingivally from the interproximal tooth surfaces and this is best achieved with dental floss, dental tape or an interdental brush, which penetrate subgingivally.

This patient should be encouraged to stop using the wooden points and to use one of the more effective methods. It is unlikely that this amount of damage could be caused by the sticks alone and it is probable that her diet has an excessive acid content. This should be investigated and the patient counselled accordingly.

**100** (a) Difficulties with oral hygiene because of the physical presence of the fraenae. Soreness due to damage during brushing to the non-keratinised mucosa overlying the fraenum. Some would claim that the fraenum exerts a pull on the gingival margin leading to the type of recession seen in the illustration. This pull is most likely secondary to the recession.
(b) This type of area is best cleaned with a single tuft or interspace type brush. If the area is too sore for brushing then a chemical antiplaque agent such as chlorhexidine gluconate could be used.
(c) Careful cleaning of the area to remove all surface deposits of plaque and calculus. Apply a desensitiser such as a fluoride varnish if the dentine is sensitive. A frenectomy may help access for cleaning. This area is not suitable for a laterally repositioned flap as there is no suitable adjacent site from which to move the tissue. A free gingival graft is a possibility.
(d) The free gingival graft together with a vestibular deepening is the only procedure which would reliably give greater depth and improve access for cleaning.

**101** (a) Bohn's nodules. These are epithelial remnants, usually of the dental lamina, which become cystic and filled with sebaceous material.
(b) They are very common, although they often go unnoticed and accurate prevalence data are hard to obtain. Probably approximately 60% of babies have one or more of these lesions but they are seldom seen in the abundance shown in this baby.
(c) Masterful inactivity with reassurance of the mother! They undergo spontaneous resolution a few months after birth.

**102** The universal curette is sharp all the way round the toe and on both sides. In addition, universal curettes can be used in all areas of the mouth on all tooth surfaces, the face of the blade is at 90° to the shank, and the instrument is curved in one plane only—the blade curves up but not to the side.

In contrast, Gracey curettes have only one cutting edge and are area-specific, i.e. a set of instruments is required to scale or root plane the whole mouth, each instrument being designed to be used on specific surfaces of specific groups of teeth. The face of the blade is at 70° to the shank so that when the instrument is in use the shank is parallel to the tooth surface and the blade is at 70° to the tooth surface (the most efficient angle for the removal of deposits). At the same time the non-sharpened side of the blade is in contact with the soft tissue wall of the pocket thus minimising trauma. Finally the blade is curved in two planes—upwards and to the side.

Gracey curettes are especially useful when removing deposits in deep pockets or other areas difficult to access, such as furcations.

**103** The condition is desquamative gingivitis. This is merely a general descriptive term and does not constitute an accurate diagnosis. Careful questioning and examination of the patient, particularly with regard to drug history, skin rashes and involvement of other mucous membranes, may suggest the nature of underlying disease and the presence of a white lacework pattern elsewhere in the mouth would indicate a diagnosis of lichen planus. Nealy all cases, however, should be subjected to biopsy which will reveal any serious underlying condition such as pemphigoid (which may cause blindness if there is ocular involvement) or pemphigus, which is a life-threatening condition. In any case of doubt the patient should be referred to an appropriate physician.

Local treatment should consist of removal of deposits and careful oral hygiene. This may prove painful for the patient to carry out effectively in which case a chlorhexidine mouthwash should be prescribed. This may be diluted with water if neat mouthwash is uncomfortable. If this regime does not produce a satisfactory result, a local steroid cream such as fluocinolone acetonide (either as 1:10 or 1:4 dilution depending on the severity of the condition) should be prescribed. This should be applied to the affected gingival tissues by a closely fitting soft splint which should be well extended into the sulci. The patient should be shown where in the splint to place the cream. The splint(s) should be worn for 15 minutes twice per day. The lesions usually show an improvement within a few weeks but it may take some months before the tissues are completely comfortable. Relapses may be treated by further short-term therapy until symptoms are relieved.

**104** (i) It is less invasive. (ii) Provides information about change at the histological level and is therefore potentially more sensitive. (iii) It is more objective than traditional indices. (iv) When used in screening it has the potential to identify groups 'at risk' from future disease activity. (v) It has the ability to identify disease activity as it is occurring and *potentially* before damage results. It therefore facilitates early diagnosis. Current methods of diagnosis identify only 'historical disease'. (vi) The sensitivity and specificity of such tests in correctly diagnosing disease are far better than traditional methods. The best of the conventional methods is bleeding on probing and that is reported to identify only 30–40% of sites undergoing active disease.

**105** (a) The procedure that has been carried out is a free gingival graft, presumably to prevent further recession occurring labial to 41. The graft is excessively long for this purpose and has healed, as all such grafts do, to a paler colour than the surrounding tissue.
(b) The stages involved in the technique of free gingival grafting are as follows: (i) Select a donor site. This is usually most conveniently situated in the palate. If not adjacent to the gingival margin, it will be necessary to take an impression in order to construct a pack retention plate for use during the postoperative period.(ii) Obtain anaesthesia at donor and recipient sites. (iii) Prepare a bed for the graft by incising at the muco-gingival junction and exposing the periosteum by sharp dissection in an apical direction. (iv) Prepare a template of the operative site (this can conveniently be done by using the sterile card around which the suture is wrapped). (v) This is transferred to the palate. The periphery of the graft is marked by pricking around the edge of the template with a suitable instrument such as a sickle scaler. (vi) The graft, about 2mm thick and as even as possible, is removed by sharp dissection. (If using a wide-bore sucker, loss of the graft via the sucker is an embarrassing possibility. This can be avoided by inserting a suture through the graft before it is finally removed, or covering the end of the sucker with a gauze square). (vii) The graft is placed on the donor site and finally trimmed. It is then sutured into position at its coronal and lateral borders only and pressed firmly into position using damp gauze to prevent the formation of a blood clot on its deep surface. This would interfere with nutrition of the graft during the time before blood vessels grow into it to develop a new circulation.
(viii) Donor and recipient sites are dressed with a periodontal dressing and the patient instructed in postoperative care, particularly in the importance of not pulling the lip forward to look at the postoperative site. Both wounds will usually need to be dressed for 2 weeks, after which the sutures may be removed.

**106** (a) Chronic periapical periodontitis from a non-vital pulp, or a lateral periodontal abscess (lateral suppurative periodontitis).
(b) (i) A pulp test, although if only one canal of a multi-rooted tooth was non-vital, it would be possible to elicit a positive response from a tooth with periapical periodontitis. (ii) A periapical radiograph showing the crestal and apical areas. The distribution of the bone loss might suggest a cause. It may also be helpful to place a guttapercha point into the pocket prior to exposing the radiograph. This may indicate the origin of the lesion, apical or lateral. (iii) Probing depths for this tooth and other suspect teeth. Although periodontal disease may be site-specific, it is usual for more than one tooth to be affected.
(c) One could assume infection by pyogenic organisms, but most periodontal abscesses are mixed infections. Entry of organisms into the connective tissues adjacent to the pocket is the most likely cause. Entry is usually via microulceration of the pocket lining. Older readers will remember the suggestion that foreign bodies, such as fish bones, fruit pips or even toothbrush bristles, might be responsible. Although this is theoretically possible, it is rarely seen. Suppuration may follow root planing, when organisms and/or calculus may be inadvertently pushed through the pocket lining into the connective tissues, during instrumentation. It is often claimed that suppuration may be caused by blockage of a pocket. Most periodontal abscesses are draining through a pocket when first seen.
(d) Drainage of the pus by extracting the tooth, root planing, surgical incision into a fluctuant lesion, use of hot salt-water mouthbaths to encourage further drainage, further root planing, with chlorhexidine irrigation as necessary. In the long term, surgical exposure of the area may be necessary to permit effective debridement.

**107** (a) Artefactual damage to upper buccal and labial attached and unattached gingiva.
(b) Identify the cause if possible—this may require extensive and prolonged history taking. In this case it was self-inflicted injury due to excessive toothbrushing. Substitute chemical oral hygiene measures (chlorhexidine mouthwash) for mechanical measures for a period of 3 weeks. This may both relieve the condition and confirm the diagnosis. Prescribe antibiotics to prevent secondary infection. Advise the patient's physician of your findings.

**108** The improvement of the patient's gingival state followed removal of all sub- and supragingival deposits and instruction of the patient in thorough plaque removal including twice daily use of a solution of 0.1% chlorhexidine delivered by a pulsed oral irrigator. Such irrigation permits penetration of the antibacterial agent subgingivally to an extent which is not possible with the use of mouthwashes or conventional mechanical plaque-removal agents. This case illustrates the importance of treating even moderately severe drug-induced gingival hyperplasia by conservative means before performing gingival surgery with its attendant risks.

**109** The lesion is probably a cotton wool roll 'burn' caused by a cotton wool roll having been placed in the buccal sulcus during preparation of the cavity, and being removed dry after it had stuck to the soft tissues. Such damage is avoided by thoroughly wetting the roll before removal. A possible alternative cause would be damage due to oil of cloves.

**110** (a) Habitual cheek biting. This appearance contrasts with the linear hyperkeratinised appearance seen in the mucosa from chronic trauma due to parafunctional activity such as nocturnal bruxism. It is more generalised with petechial haemorrhages.
(b) Advise the patient to discontinue the habit. In severe cases, an occlusal guard may be necessary; its presence not only helps to prevent the trauma but serves as a reminder to the child not to persist with the habit.

**111** Stippling. When one looks at a histological section of gingiva, the epithelium is seen to be of uneven thickness and prolongations of epithelium extend into the underlying connective tissue. These are known as rete pegs. When serial sections are examined, it becomes apparent that each rete peg is part of a rete ridge which extends through many serial sections rather like an inverted range of mountains. Moreover, there are many such ridges and where they cross each other the gingival surface is dimpled. This is a stipple. It is interesting to note that dental folk lore still teaches that stippling is caused by the free gingival collagen fibres being attached to the epithelium *between* the rete pegs, thus pulling down the surface. This is quite wrong—the indentation or stipple is always in the middle of the rete peg.

**112** (a) Active sites not responding to non-surgical therapy. Chemical plaque control is indicated because of physical difficulties or handicap. The topography of the lesion makes mechanical oral hygiene ineffective. The patient has a fixed restoration such as a bridge which limits the access for mechanical oral hygiene.
(b) A pulsed oral irrigator is able to deliver a chemical solution subgingivally, to a limited extent. This is not possible with rinsing. The pulsed delivery of the oral irrigator improves the effectiveness of any chemical adjunct, therefore lower concentrations of the chemical may be used. The irrigator is able to deliver large volumes of a chemical solution and this again increases the efficiency. Studies show that irrigation is more efficient than rinsing with regard to reductions in plaque levels. When chlorhexidine is used in an oral irrigator at a lower concentration than is used in a mouthwash staining is less.
(c) Bacteraemia has been reported, and care is therefore needed in patients at risk from endocarditis. Abscess formation has been reported. These devices involve water and electricity and their use in bathrooms must follow the usual guidelines for electrical safety. They are expensive, messy and time-consuming to use.
(d) Supragingival, high pressure. Plastic subgingival, low pressure. Needle-type subgingival, low pressure.

**113** (a) A replaced flap (could have been developed by a crevicular incision alone, or in combination with an inverse bevel incision, as in the modified Widman flap approach).
(b) (i) Surgical access to root surface and alveolar bone. (ii) Pocket reduction in cases of moderate (5–6mm) and severe (7+mm pocketing) chronic periodontitis which has been uncontrolled by satisfactory local measures. Particularly appropriate around anterior teeth where minimum recession is required for cosmetic reasons.
(c) Compared to non-surgical treatment, the replaced flap allows direct visual and mechanical access for root debridement or amputation, odontoplasty, osteoplasty and regeneration procedures.
   Compared to gingivectomy and ARF, the replaced flap is less intrusive, heals mainly by primary intention, gives less postoperative discomfort and much less gingival recession. If there is sufficient horizontal length of incision, vertical relieving incisions are not usually required.

**114** The patient is taking cyclosporin, a selective immunosuppressant which prevents graft rejection. One of the unwanted effects of this drug is gingival overgrowth which is illustrated in this picture.
   Approximately 30% of dentate organ transplant patients medicated with cyclosporin experience significant gingival overgrowth. This requires mechanical plaque control. Full liaison with the patient's physician is essential in the management of these patients. The

patient is immunosuppressed and most physicians request antibiotic cover prior to any dental procedures (i.e .gingival surgery) which can result in a bacteraemia. Amoxycillin 3g orally is the drug of choice. If the patient is allergic to penicillin, then clindamycin 600mg should be given. Erythromycin is contra-indicated in patients taking cyclosporin, since it reduces the hepatic metabolism of the immunosuppressant. This causes an increase in plasma concentrations of cyclosporin and thus an increase in the renal toxicity of the drug. Nearly all renal organ transplant patients are taking prednisolone (a corticosteroid) and thus require steroid cover prior to surgery.

Recurrence of cyclosporin-induced gingival overgrowth is a problem in organ transplant patients. Unlike phenytoin and nifedipine, there is no alternative medication for the patient to change to. Thorough attention to oral hygiene and regular maintenance programmes are required for these patients.

**115** Common faults found in porcelain jacket crowns include excessive subgingival extension, marginal overhangs and deficiencies and excess interproximal bulk of porcelain which impinges on the interdental space. In addition, patients are often not instructed in proper home care after crowns have been fitted. It is important that the cement lute is kept free of plaque by proper use of toothbrush and floss or tape.

Before the crowns are replaced it is important that gingival health is restored and the level of the gingival margin stabilised. Radiographs should be taken to check for the presence of periapical disease. The existing crowns should be removed and an impression of the preparations recorded. Temporary crowns are fitted immediately and on the model, laboratory-made acrylic crowns are constructed to replace them as soon as possible. The periodontitis is treated by scaling, plaque control, root planing and if necessary periodontal surgery to obtain gingival health and a satisfactory contour. The preparations can then be modified so that their margins lie just beneath the gingival margin and permanent crowns are constructed.

**116** (a) (i) Inadequate tongue protection and moisture control. (ii) Instrumentation being used without rubber gloves.
(b) (i) Electrosurgery should be used for small areas of soft tissue removal only.
(ii) Prolonged contact with the soft tissues should be avoided. (iii) Bone contact must be avoided since this will produce necrosis. (iv) When taking impressions, the procedure should be used for haemorrhage control only; it should not be used for 'troughing'.
(v) Non-metallic instruments only should be used in the operating field. (vi) Contact with metallic restorations must be avoided.

**117** The long-term complications of gingivectomy are likely to be the recurrence of gingival inflammation by hyperplasia. These may be due to:(i) inadequate pocket removal; (ii) failure to maintain oral hygiene; and (iii) continuation of drug therapy (e.g. epanutin).

Other complications may be root sensitivity, root caries and poor aesthetics. This is particularly true if the patient is still using medication, e.g. epanutin (which may have been the cause of hyperplasia initially), or if the patient has failed or is unable to maintain good plaque control. Alternatively, pockets may not have been completely removed at the time of surgery, either because the gingivectomy was insufficiently radical or because interdental craters existed which were inadequately curetted or could have been more satisfactorily managed by flap surgery to permit better access.

**118** (a) Type 1: non-resorbable, e.g. expanded polytetrafluoroethylene (PTFE) fibre membranes.Type 2: resorbable membranes, e.g. cross-linked collagen membranes.

(b) One week for removal of flap sutures (these may be left in longer). Weekly or 2-weekly review for oral hygiene instruction (OHI) and maintenance of a high standard of plaque control. At 6 weeks the membrane is removed.

(c) Unpredictable resorption times.

(d) (i) Class I and II furcation involvements. (ii) Infrabony defects (those involving vertical bone loss). Defects should have 2 or 3 walls. (iii) Crescentic bone loss and dehiscence defects. (iv) For infill of periapical granuloma/cyst defects with bone. (v) For ridge augmentation prior to construction of a prosthesis. (vi) To maintain alveolar height after tooth extraction. (vii) To augment the placement of osseointegrated implants (pre- or post-placement of implants) or in the salvage of failing implants. (viii) Oro-antro fistulas (with a maxillary sinus lift).

**119** (a) Fordyce spots.

(b) Ectopic sebaceous glands.

(c) No treatment is required other than reassurance of the patient that the lesion is of no consequence.

**120**

| Gingival tissues | Healthy | Diseased |
| --- | --- | --- |
| Colour | Pink | Red-bluish red |
| Size | Normal | Enlarged |
| Shape | Knife edge (scalloped) | Blunt |
| Plaque deposits | Minimal | Definite plaque present |
| Gentle probing | No bleeding | Bleeding |

Clinical loss of attachment is identified by a true pocket, the base of which is apical to the cement–enamel junction. This may be confirmed by radiographic assessment which will demonstrate the level of alveolar bone.

**121** (a) (i) Erosion of dietary origin. (ii) Erosion of reflux origin: hiatus hernia; alcoholism; achlorhydria; dietary reflux activity. (iii) Combined erosion etiology. (iv) Erosion with superimposed parafunction. (v) Chronic gingivitis with some direct trauma.

(b) (i) Plaque control. (ii) Diet and reflux investigation followed by advice and further care. (iii) Complete upper overdenture prosthesis. This would perform a dual function, providing both an improvement in aesthetics and giving some protection to the eroded upper teeth. (iv) Fluoride application to the supporting teeth daily. (v) Study cast to ensure that the preventive precautions which have been taken have been effective.

It should be remembered that subsequent reconstruction with fixed restorations would be most unwise if this erosive problem continued. It would be particularly difficult to reconstruct this patient because of the lack of supragingival coronal tissue in the upper arch.

**122** This condition is chronic gingivitis and in this particular case, in view of the swelling, the term' chronic hyperplastic gingivitis' could be used.

The clinical features are: (i) redness; (ii) swelling or oedema; (iii) loss of gingival stippling; (iv) bleeding on minor trauma such as toothbrushing or gentle probing with a blunt instrument; and (v) no loss of attachment.

The most important local factor is, in the first instance, inadequate plaque control in these areas. Aggravating factors could include a poor lip seal consequent on incompetent lips or mouth-breathing.

**123**

| | Lateral periodontal abscess | Apical Abscess |
|---|---|---|
| Vitality of tooth | Usually vital | Non-vital (but beware multi-rooted teeth) |
| Pain | Less severe than apical abscess | Very severe usually |
| Discharge | Through pocket | Usually over apex but may be at gingival margin |
| Swelling | More gingivally | Over apex |
| Area of maximum tenderness | More gingivally | Over apex |
| Timing | Usually swelling before pain | Usually pain before swelling |
| Tenderness to percussion | Usually, not very | Yes, very |
| Pocketing | Yes | Not necessarily |
| History of trauma or previous filling | Not necessarily | Usually |
| Previous symptoms of pulpitis | Not necessarily | Often |
| Appearance on X-ray | Marginal bone loss visible | May be apical rarefaction |

**124** The dental hygienist must either: (i) have completed additional training in local infiltration analgesia and gained a certificate in the administration of local infiltration analgesia; (ii) have gained the Certificate of Proficiency in Dental Hygiene more than 12 months after the coming into force of the Dental Auxiliaries (Amendment) Regulations 1991; or (iii) hold the Certificate of Proficiency as a Dental Therapist in addition to the Certificate of Proficiency in Dental Hygiene. When appointing a dental hygienist the employer should always ask to see proof of the hygienist's current registration with the General Dental Council and, if appropriate, the certificate of administration of local infiltration analgesia issued by a School of Dental Hygiene and signed by the Director or Deputy Director of the School.

**125** (a) Diagnosis: (i) Chronic adult periodontitis.
(ii) Direct gingival trauma with some parafunctional activity at night.
(iii) Muscle dysfunction.
(iv) Overclosure.
(b) Treatment plan: (i) Oral hygiene instruction involving the use of an interspace brush and dental tape in areas of gingival recession.
(ii) Provisional removable appliances to re-establish the correct vertical relation, provide posterior support and restore anterior guidance. Upper and lower removable appliances will be required.
(iii) Counselling with regard to muscle dysfunction.
(iv) Review to reassess the periodontal status and symptomatology prior to definitive appliances in cobalt–chromium alloy with resin-functional surfaces.

Consideration could be given to a combined oral surgery and orthodontic approach directed towards a defined restorative outcome. The latter approach would only be justifiable in the event of the periodontal disease being adequately treated. It would have the advantage of establishing anterior guidance without resorting to a bulky maxillary removable appliance.

**126** Brown extrinsic discolouration of the teeth due to the precipitation of dietary chromogens onto the tooth surface by chlorhexidine. Chlorhexidine is a dicationic bis-biguanide antiseptic which adsorbs to the tooth surface where it can interact with dietary polyphenols which are negatively charged.
Side-effects: (i) Unpleasant taste. (ii) Taste disturbance. (iii) Mucosal burning sensations. (iv) Mucosal erosions. (v) Extrinsic staining of the dorsum of the tongue. (vi) Increased supragingival calculus formation. (vii) Unilateral or bilateral parotid swelling.

Chlorhexidine should not be placed in the auditory canal since in the presence of a perforation in the tympanic membrane middle ear deafness may ensue.

**127** (a) (i) Haemangioma.
(ii) Viral wart.
(iii) Peripheral giant cell lesion.
(b) This young girl had viral warts on the fingers of her right hand. The histopathology was consistent with a diagnosis of molluscum contagiosum, a form of wart thought to be of viral origin. A definitive diagnosis can only be made following biopsy.
Histopathologically, the lesions are characterised by 'molluscum contagiosum cells' which are large and spongy in appearance and often have a 'glassy cytoplasm'. **127B** and **127C** demonstrate viral warts of the scalp and gingival infection with the same virus.

**128** Diagnosis: acute necrotising ulcerative gingivitis.

Clinical features: localised or generalised destruction of the interdental papillae and marginal gingiva. In the acute stage of the condition, ulcerative necrosis and sloughing may be evident. In non-HIV patients, the destruction would normally be confined to the papillary gingivae.

Treatment: (i) Debridement and scaling to remove calculus from crown and root surfaces. (ii) Individualised oral hygiene instruction and motivation. (iii) In cases of pronounced lymphadenitis or severe tissue destruction consider chemotherapeutic agent; metronizadole 200mg three times daily for 5 days or penicillin (phenoxymethyl penicillin) 250mg four times daily for 5 days. (iv) Recall after 5 days and institute frequent maintenance regime.

**129** Assuming that the patient does not have blood dyscrasia, haemangioma or is not taking medication likely to cause an increased bleeding time, the most likely complication during gingivectomy is excessive bleeding caused by inflammation due to inadequate presurgical therapy. This, in turn, is likely to lead to premature loss of local anaesthetic solution from the tissues and increasing pain. It is very important, therefore, that plaque and gingivitis are well controlled and that ample time is allowed to achieve resolution prior to surgery, which may mean that gingivectomy is not required after all. Anaesthesia should be achieved by infiltration close to, or actually into the tissue to be excised, using an agent which gives adequately prolonged anaesthesia and contains a vasoconstrictor.

**130** The patient has generalised periodontal disease and the initial cause of the pain was a lateral periodontal abscess associated with 11, as can be seen in the illustration. Questioning revealed, however, that the patient had tried to deal with this herself by applying cotton wool soaked in an undiluted household antiseptic agent to the area. This is in contradiction to the manufacturer's instructions, which advise considerable dilution when the product is used as a mouthwash. The application has caused extensive soft tissue damage with considerable sloughing of the epithelium.

The condition can be dealt with by advising the patient not to use any more of her self-prescribed medication. Discomfort can be eased by the use of a lignocaine gel. The lateral periodontal abscess should be drained either through the pocket or via an incision. The root surface should be rendered free from plaque and calculus by subgingival instrumentation.

**131** The patient has gingivitis modified (i.e. made more florid) by her pregnancy. The correct treatment is to remove all deposits professionally and to show her how to remove plaque at home twice daily. This is particularly important interdentally and below the gum margin. The use of dental floss or tape and the Bass technique of brushing would be appropriate in her case.

**132** (a) Papillon-Lefèvre syndrome (hyperkeratosis palmoplantaris and periodontoclasia). This is an autosomal recessive condition with parental consanguinity in about 40% of cases. The primary teeth erupt normally but the gingivae then swell and spontaneous haemorrhage occurs. The parents may notice a marked halitosis. Destruction of the periodontium appears to accompany the development of the palmar and plantar hyperkeratosis.
(b) Plaque control and root planing. Any unsaveable teeth should be extracted. Long-term antibiotic therapy (usually with tetracycline) has been tried but with generally disappointing results. Unfortunately most teeth are usually lost by the mid-teens.
(c) Trauma; juvenile periodontitis; Papillon-Lefèvre syndrome; histiocytosis X; neutropenia; hypophosphatasia; acatalasia; Chediak–Higashi syndrome; acrodynia; leukaemia.

**133** (a) A constant force probe.
(b) It has a spring-loaded mechanism which causes the probe to 'break' at a pre-set force (usually 20–25g) which is, therefore, the maximum force that can be applied. It has been shown that forces in excess of 25g can cause a conventional probe to penetrate the tissues at the base of periodontal pockets thus exaggerating their depth as well as causing discomfort to the patient. It is difficult if not impossible consistently to apply a force of 25g with a conventional probe. The constant force probe is especially useful in experimental and epidemiological investigations, in which it reduces examiner error.

**134** This is a typical case of pipe-smoker's keratosis. The white appearance is due to an increase in the thickness of the keratin layer of the hard palate brought about by chemical and thermal irritation. The red spots are the openings of the ducts of minor salivary glands.

The condition may be potentlally malignant and the patient should be advised to stop smoking. If this proves impossible, an acrylic plate can be constructed to cover the palate for use during smoking.

**135** (a) Rapid local changes in pressure as the negative pressure bubbles implode. Removal of root surface deposits. Disruption of micro-organisms. Improved healing following use.

(b) Prolonged aerosol. The high frequency vibrations cause temporary shifts in hearing which may be permanent in dental personnel. The electromagnetic emissions may interfere with pacemakers. The procedure may be painful in some patients. It may damage crown and bridgework.

(c) It would be unwise to use the ultrasonic scaler in patients with Hepatitis B as the aerosol may be a risk to subsequent patients (assuming that the dental personnel are protected by vaccination). There would also be a risk of dental personnel contracting Hepatitis C. It should also be avoided in HIV-positive patients as they may be at risk of lung infections from organisms in the aerosol.

(d) Acoustic micro-streaming.

**136** (a) No, it is the mandibular fraenum that is associated with recession. This is most likely due to the lack of underlying labial bone that occurs in the mandible. The maxillary fraenum is usually well supported by bone.

(b) It is frequently associated with pocketing due to the increased retention of dental plaque. It may also be associated with a mid-line diastema, as in the illustration.

(c) A frenectomy, usually performed using local analgesia. Incisions are made in attached gingiva alongside the fraenum down to bone. The fraenum is grasped with forceps and an incision made along the mucogingival junction to join the two lateral incisions. Using a periosteal elevator the fraenum is then raised and removed. A deep suture is placed at the mucogingival junction and a periodontal dressing placed.

**137** A case of gingival hyperplasia caused by cyclosporin is illustrated. The patient was treated by simple gingivectomy under general anaesthesia. Because of the risk of excessive haemorrhage in extreme cases such as this, the anaesthetist should be advised of the need to inject a vasoconstrictor into the tissues and cross-matched blood should be available. Hyperplasia may also be plaque-induced, hereditary or caused by epanutin or nifedipine. Normally treatment is by gingivectomy under local analgesia, unless there has been bone loss, when flap surgery may be indicated.

**138** (a) Erythema multiforme. The severe form involves genital and ocular ulceration and is called Stevens–Johnson Syndrome.

(b) The most common causes involve hypersensitivity reactions to certain drugs and some are thought to be of viral aetiology, e.g. previous infection with the herpes simplex virus. In some cases the cause is unknown.

(c) The histology of this condition is very variable and the diagnosis should be made clinically. Classically, there are vesiculobullous-type eruptions, erythematous and oedematous areas. Skin lesions, called 'target ' or 'iris' lesions, are diagnostic (**138C**) and there may be a haemorrhagic circumoral crusting.

(d) The most likely aetiology in this case is a combination of extreme stress and drug therapy. There was no history of herpes simplex.

**139** (a) Herpes simplex virus (HSV).

(b) The herpes viruses, an important group of large DNA viruses which includes: herpes simplex virus 1 (HSV-1); herpes simplex virus 2 (HSV-2); varicella-zoster virus (VZV); Epstein-Barr virus (EPV); cytomegalovirus CMV); and human herpes virus 6 (HHV6).

(c) Herpes simplex typically persists in the body after the primary infection (to become a latent infection), and may subsequently be reactivated to cause local recurrence of clinical lesions. In the case of oral HSV infections, the virus commonly remains latent in the trigeminal ganglion and, on reactivation by stimuli such as exposure to trauma or the sun, travels along the neural axon to reach the epithelium. The recurrent outbreaks typically appear as 'cold sores' or herpes labialis.

(d) HSV infection can be diagnosed by direct examination of biopsy material or smears (stained with specific monoclonal antibody reagents), laboratory culture of the virus, or by demonstration of increasing antibody levels in the blood.

(e) For the dentist, infection of the finger can lead to the development of an herpetic whitlow. More severe infections can also occur in some patients, especially those who are immunocompromised, including eye infections, HSV encephalitis and neonatal herpes. Genital herpes infections are common and can be caused by either of the HS viruses, although HSV-2 is found more frequently in this situation.

(f) Severe cases of primary herpetic stomatitis may be treated with oral and topically applied acyclovir, together with symptomatic treatment. Recurrent herpetic infections are not normally treated with acyclovir unless they occur in immunocompromised patients, or there is a history of severe and extensive lesions.

**140** Differential diagnosis: oral contraceptive-induced gingival pigmentation; gingival ephylis (freckle).

On questioning, the patient was aware of the lesion having appeared around the time that she had begun taking the oral contraceptive. She was taking a combination contraceptive containing gestodene and ethinyloestradiol. Oral pigmentation has been reported to be associated with oestrodiol-based preparations which are believed to have a stimulatory effect on the secretion of pituitary malanocyte-stimulating hormone. There are no reports of similar occurrences with progesterone-only medications, and the pigmentation does not resolve completely on cessation of the medication.

The lesion should be well documented and, if possible, photographed for reference. The patient should be regularly reviewed initially and if there is any indication of change in the lesion, it should be biopsied. The condition is totally benign and of little clinical relevance, apart from the fact that it is important to distinguish it from melanoma or an underlying systemic condition (e.g. Addison's disease).

**141** Upper first premolars usually have two root canals, one buccal and one palatal. This is reflected in a longitudinal depression on the mesial surface extending from the enamel–cement junction to the apex that is known as the 'canine groove'. If bone loss occurs interproximally plaque control becomes impossible because the patient cannot clean in the groove and disease is likely to progress. Postoperative care:

(a) In the first week will depend on whether a periodontal dressing has been placed or not. If it has, the patient should be advised to avoid the area when cleaning the teeth and to take care when eating. If no periodontal dressing has been placed the patient should be advised to rinse the area for two minutes twice per day with 0·2% chlorhexidine.

(b) In the longer term, interproximal plaque control should be by means of an interdental brush which will keep the groove free of plaque.

**142** The lesion is a cementoma or periapical cemental dysplasia. These are symptomless and begin as areas of radiolucency involving the periodontal ligament spaces in the apical region of teeth. They have a strong radiological resemblance to apical infection and many teeth have been extracted or root filled because of mistaken diagnosis. The teeth most commonly affected are lower incisors.

The lesion starts as a circumscribed replacement of bone by fibrous tissue. Later this fibrous tissue undergoes calcification and in this mature state the cementoma is strikingly radiopaque. The one shown in the photograph is semi-mature with islands and strands of calcification. Cementomata are entirely benign and need no treatment.

**143** (a) (i) Lack of success in providing a conventional restoration for the missing teeth. It is generally agreed that osseointegrated implants should be the last line of treatment which may be provided, if all other approaches fail. (ii) Healthy mucosal tissues. Mucosal lesions such as denture-induced stomatitis, hyperplasia, candidiasis or other lesions can be treated prior to implant placement. This patient has denture-induced stomatitis. (iii) Sound bony morphology. Bony lesions such as retained roots, impacted teeth or cysts must be corrected first and time allowed for healing prior to the implant placement. The ridge thickness, density and morphology must also be sufficient to permit placement of the implant.
(iv) Sufficient space to place the implants. A single tooth replacement implant will require a minimum of 7mm between adjacent teeth and 7mm of bone depth. Multiple partial replacements should ideally have a minimum of 3 osseointegrated abutments for adequate support.
(b) Provided the patient can withstand the necessary surgery, there are very few general medical contra-indications to implant treatment. Osseointegrated implants have been provided for patients with such diverse medical conditions as diabetes, arthritis, cardiac and vascular problems, as well as for those receiving long-term steroid therapy, with no long-term adverse effects. Patients with psychiatric problems can present some difficulties in long-term management. The local medical conditions which require treatment prior to implant placement are indicated in part (a) of this question.
(c) Oral hygiene advice, including appropriate care of the existing denture. Dietary advice, to reduce the high caries rate, including possible home topical fluoride therapy. A check of the existing denture and modification if it is contributing to the present problems. Long-term decision on the most appropriate definitive restoration.
(d) The definitive prosthesis will depend upon the patient's wishes and the expertise of the operator. A well-designed acrylic denture of the Every type should be maintainable with good oral hygiene. A metal-based denture will allow more flexibility of design, less tissue coverage, improved retention, support and stability. A fixed bridge would be possible and would be the most appropriate restoration for this patient.

**144** The woman is preparing 'pan'. This consists of betel nut cut in half, dipped in slaked lime and wrapped in tobacco leaves. The lesion seen in **144B** is hyperkeratosis caused by the patient habitually holding the pan between his cheek and gum. It is potentially premalignant and the patient should be advised to discontinue the habit. The area should be inspected at monthly intervals until it has disappeared. Any areas of induration or reddening should be examined by incisional biopsy.

**145** (a) Probing depth is the depth to which a periodontal probe may be inserted into a periodontal pocket, measured from the gingival margin.
(b) Pocket depth is the depth from the gingival margin to the base of a periodontal pocket. Because a probe can penetrate diseased tissue and the junctional epithelium at the base of a pocket the probing depth may be deeper than the pocket depth.

(c) Loss of attachment is defined as the distance from the amelocemental junction to the base of the pocket. It is calculated by measuring from the gingival margin to the base of the pocket and then measuring from the gingival margin to the amelocemental junction. Subtracting the second measurement from the first gives loss of attachment. Locating the amelocemental junction by purely tactile means can be difficult and is complicated by deposits on the tooth surface and margins of restorations. If recession has occurred and the amelocemental junction is visible measurements are easier.

**146** (a) Childhood hypophosphatasia. This condition is hereditary and involves deficiency of the liver/bone/kidney (L/B/K) isoenzyme of alkaline phosphatase (ALP). There are four forms of hypophosphatasia, perinatal/lethal, infantile, childhood and adult, according to age of presentation. The two former types are often fatal and thought to be autosomal recessive, the latter are milder and thought to be autosomal dominant.
(b) Confirmatory tests should show low levels of serum ALP and raised plasma levels of pyridoxal-5-phosphate (vitamin $B_6$) and inorganic pyrophosphate. Urinary levels of phosphoethanolamine are raised in a 24-hour sample. These 3 substances are substrates of ALP and therefore a deficiency in ALP causes their levels to rise.
 The provisional diagnosis in this case was made from a 0·14μl sample of gingival fluid which demonstrated very low ALP levels when compared to an age-matched control.
(c) It is thought that the low serum ALP causes a defect in cementum mineralisation. The resultant cementum hypoplasia/ aplasia leads to poor attachment and tooth loss.
(d) Management should include proper genetic counselling and investigation of other family members. The condition usually is limited to anterior deciduous and occasionally permanent teeth. Treatment involves regular periodontal maintenance.

**147** (a) 3-walled (or combined 2- and 3-walled) infrabony defect arising from an infrabony pocket.
(b) It is detected and diagnosed by a comparison of probing pocket depths or attachment levels with radiographic examination by either bitewings or long cone paralleling technique. The extent of penetration of the probe clinically can be assessed on the radiograph to determine whether or not the base of the pocket is below the level of the adjacent alveolar bone crest—hence infrabony. Alternatively, under local analgesia, transgingival probing of the underlying alveolar bone topography will often reveal the extent and type of bone loss.
(c) (i) Non-surgical management. This may involve root planing by conventional or ultrasonic scaling, sometimes supplemented by local chemical irrigation. (ii) Replaced flap without osteoplasty (removal of some non-supporting bone). (iii) Replaced flap with osteoplasty and, occasionally, osteoectomy (removal of some supporting bone) to reduce the infrabony defect and improve flap margin adaptation. (iv) Replaced flap with bone or alloplast graft. (v) Replaced flap with guided tissue regeneration procedure. (vi) Apic lly repositioned flap, with or without osteoplasty or osteoectomy.

**148** Within the gingival tissues, the epithelium becomes thinner, less keratinised and there is an increase in cell density. The interface between the epithelium and connective tissue changes from a ridge-type to a papilla-type with increasing age. Within the periodontal ligament, the fibre and cellular components decrease and the structure of the ligament becomes more irregular with increasing age. Other changes include a reduction in cell density and mitotic activity, a reduction in organic matrix production and loss of acid mucopolysaccharide. There is no change in the width of the periodontal ligament with increasing age; this factor is governed by the occlusal loading. Cementum formation continues throughout life and the increase in width with age is most marked in the apical region. A slight increase in remodelling of cementum also occurs with age and is characterised by areas of resorption and apposition. Alveolar bone shows changes with age that include an increase in the number of interstitial lamellae, producing dense interdental septa, and a decrease in the number of cells in the osteogenic layer of the cribriform plate. With increasing age, the periodontal surfaces of the alveolar bone become jagged and collagen fibres show a less regular insertion into bone.

There is controversy over the relationship between ageing and attachment loss. Animal studies suggest that ageing is associated with a gradual, physiological recession of the gingival tissues with an apical migration of the junctional epithelium. This idea would support the theory of continuous passive eruption, which proposes that gingival recession occurs as a result of occlusal migration of the teeth. The migration compensates for occlusal wear. Subsequent studies have shown that occlusal movement of the teeth is not necessarily associated with apical migration of the junctional epithelium. There is thus little evidence to support the physiological apical migration of the junctional epithelium with age.

Age changes in the periodontium do not appear to be significant factors in determining either the response of the periodontal tissue to plaque or treatment.

**149** (i) The crown restorations are being reconstructed in the presence of gingival disease. There is evidence of poor plaque control and chronic gingivitis elsewhere in the mouth. (ii) Prepared crown margins are being taken into a subgingival area where it will be impossible to detect adequately whether they fit well. (iii) The provisional crown restorations have exacerbated the gingival disease. (iv) The castings have been designed to give insufficient space for proximal surface porcelain and space for proximal surface cleansing. In addition the metalwork will give inadequate support to the incisal porcelain. (v) The gingival exudate and haemorrhage will prevent appropriate moisture control during cementation when the crowns are completed. This problem can be avoided by ensuring good plaque control and gingival health prior to embarking upon crown restoration. In the event of crown restorations being required to replace pre-existing restorations, plaque control should be improved initially to achieve gingival health and a surgical procedure used to establish a new stable gingival margin away from the restoration margins. Well-made and well-polished provisional crown restorations will subsequently allow reasonable aesthetics while appropriate healing takes place. Subsequent definitive crown margins should not be taken into the subgingival area.

**150** (a) Infectious mononucleosis with bilateral periocoronitis.
(b) (i) Full blood count and platelets with differential white cell count. (ii) Peripheral blood film for atypical lymphocytes. (iii) Paul–Bunnell test for heterophil antibodies or monospot test.
(c) Symptomatic: fluids; soft diet; antipyretics and analgesics; local antiseptics.
  Antibiotics may be necessary for secondary infection. However, antibiotics of the penicillin group should be avoided as they may cause a rash.

**151** The lesion is reddish and therefore fairly vascular. The most likely diagnosis is a pyogenic granuloma caused by irritation from an orthodontic appliance although the possibility of a peripheral giant cell granuloma should not be excluded. The latter however, tends to occur in older patients.

The correct treatment is to remove the lesion by excisional biopsy and subject it to histological examination. Care should be taken to remove the lesion completely, i.e. down to bone, and the wound should be dressed at weekly intervals using a periodontal dressing until it is completely epithelised. If good interdental plaque control is achieved, these steps will usually prevent recurrence.

Histologically, the pyogenic granuloma is identical with a pregnancy tumour, its main characteristics being endothelial-lined vascular spaces, immature collagen, budding endothelial cells and proliferating fibroblasts. If untreated, the pyogenic granuloma may mature in time to become a fibrous epulis.

The other dental abnormality present is fusion of 41 and 42 with production of a 'double tooth'.

**152** (a) The second premolar has already erupted and the second molar is partially erupted. Therefore, the extraction will result in tipping of the second molar mesially and will produce a poor contact with possible food packing. It is also possible that the upper first permanent molar will over-erupt.
(b) If loss of one first permanent molar is enforced then balancing and compensating extractions of the other first permanent molars should always be considered.
(c) If the space is not required for orthodontic purposes, then the optimal time for removal is when the bifurcation of the second molar has just commenced calcification. This is generally around the age of 9 to 9.5 years. The unerupted second molar then tends to move anteriorly before eruption and there is a much better chance of a reasonable contact between the second premolar and second molar. The timing is much more critical in the mandible than the maxilla.

**153** The pattern of inflammation around the gingival margins is strongly suggestive of residual subgingival calculus that is acting as a plaque-retention factor. Other reasons why inflammation persists may be that the restorations are overhanging and acting as plaque-retention factors, or that the patient's standard of plaque control is inadequate.

**154** The inflammation is due to inadequate plaque control of both gingival margins and the denture, probably because the patient was not informed of the great importance of these in preventing inflammation when the denture was provided. There is also excessive tissue coverage. The hyperplasia may have initially arisen as a result of relief of the gingival margins when the denture was made. Hobkirk and Strahan 1989) stated:
'The gingivae enlarge under all types of relief and also where there is no relief but to a much lesser extent...Partial prostheses should cover the gingival margins as little as possible but where that is unavoidable be very closely adapted to them.'

In this case the palatal gingival tissues should be returned to health before a new denture of better design is provided. Inflammation is controlled by thorough scaling and instruction in oral hygiene.

A tissue conditioner should be applied to the fitting surface of the denture which should be soaked nightly in a hypochlorite-based denture cleaner. The tissue conditioner should be replaced at intervals of 2 weeks for the first 6 weeks. After this, it may remain in place for 1 month. In favourable circumstances, gingival health should return within 3 months, at which time any areas of hyperplasia remaining may be removed by localised gingivectomy. A new denture may then be provided. This may be of a modified spoon design if acrylic or a skeleton denture if in metal.

**155** (a) Gingival veneer.

(b) (i) The veneer is indicated in cases of an unacceptable cosmetic result following perio-dontal disease and treatment, especially of upper anterior teeth. Cosmetic problems include long clinical crowns, large interdental spaces and absence of pink gingivae. (ii) Cervical sensitivity may also be reduced by wearing a veneer which can also be used to retain topical fluoride around sensitive areas. (iii) A veneer can be used to replace one or two missing anterior teeth without resorting to palatal coverage.

(iv) Application of topical steroid to areas of erosive lichen planus, benign mucous membrane pemphigoid, etc., on the labial gingivae can also be facilitated by a veneer. (v) Excessive sibilant sounds arising from anterior interdental or inter-implant spacing may be eliminated with a gingival veneer.

(c) The veneer is retained by engaging distal, horizontal undercuts on opposing sides of the anterior arch of 'elongated' teeth, and by resting on the cement–enamel junction (CEJ) ledge of these teeth. A thin salivary film achieved by a close-fitting veneer also contributes to retention.

(d) Methyl methacrylate or silicone-based materials.

**156** The instrument is a tongue scraper. These were once commonly used throughout Europe, but their use is now mainly confined to Eastern cultures. When used on a daily basis they remove debris from the dorsum of the tongue, which is a nidus for the proliferation of bacteria which are responsible for the formation of dental plaque, especially when the tongue is heavily furred.

The tongue scraper is, therefore, very useful in reducing the total microbial count of the mouth and studies have shown that plaque regrows less rapidly on teeth after cleaning when a tongue scraper is used once or twice daily on a regular basis.

If, therefore, patients have difficulty in maintaining good oral hygiene and especially if they have furred tongues, the use of a tongue scraper may well be worth trying. A teaspoon or dessert spoon (depending on the size of the patient's mouth and tongue) serves as a convenient domestic alternative.

**157** (a) Hand, foot and mouth disease.

(b) Coxsackie A virus – most commonly Coxsackie A16, but types A4, A5, A9 and A10 may also be implicated occasionally.

(c) Coxsackie A viruses belong to the group of small RNA viruses collectively known as picornaviruses. These are divided into the enteroviruses (which include Coxsackie A and B viruses, echoviruses and polioviruses) and the rhinoviruses, which are important causes of the common cold.

(d) Enteroviruses are most often spread by the oral-faecal route and can usually be isolated from faeces. Coxsackie A viruses, including those which cause hand, foot and mouth disease, may also be isolated from vesicular fluid or saliva. Some types of Coxsackie A are difficult to cultivate in conventional laboratory cell lines, but can be grown in newborn mice. Since the disease is usually mild and can be diagnosed clinically, laboratory investigations are not always necessary.

(e) No.

**158** (a) The view obtained in the upper radiograph has been obtained by 'bisecting the angle'. In this view the central ray is directed at right angles to an imaginary line that bisects the angle between the long axis of the tooth and that of the film. This results in superimposition and distortion of the true relationship between the buccal and lingual cement–enamel junctions and the buccal and lingual bone levels in the interdental spaces. This technique also, although giving accurate views of the apices of the teeth, may not show caries unless it is advanced and effectively superimposes amalgam restorations on any caries that may be beneath them.

(b) Accurate views for periodontal diagnostic purposes are obtained by conventional bitewings in cases of early bone loss. Where bone loss is more advanced the film can be turned through 90° and a 'vertical' bitewing view recorded. If periapical disease or root form needs to be examined, a paralleling method such as the long cone technique needs to be employed, such that the long axes of the tooth and the film are parallel to each other and the X-ray beam is at right angles to both.

**159** (a) Primary Sjögrens syndrome is characterised by xerostomia (dry mouth) and keratoconjunctivitis sicca (dry eyes). Secondary Sjögrens syndrome is the term used to describe those features of primary Sjögrens, plus a connective tissue disorder such as rheumatoid arthritis, systemic lupus erythematosus, polyarteritis nodosa or polymyositis.

(b) Useful investigations include salivary flow rates, Schirmer's test (tear flow rates), labial gland biopsy, sialography, salivary scintiscanning and various serological tests. The minor gland histology is of lymphoid infiltration associated with acinar atrophy and replacement fibrosis. The lymphoid infiltrate is adjacent to blood vessels and focal in nature. Serological tests include anti-Ro and anti-La antibodies (to these nuclear protein antigens), also rheumatoid factor and immunoglobulin levels (mainly IgG and IgM). The latter are useful to monitor since increasing levels may indicate development of lymphoma, a complication in 7% of Sjögrens cases.

(c) It is important to maintain a high standard of plaque control to prevent the development of cervical caries and periodontal disease. This can arise due to plaque retention within the carious cavities. Management is similar to patients who have undergone radiotherapy, i.e. dietary advice, regular scaling/polishing, fluoride therapy and if necessary artificial saliva sprays.

**160** This is a case of chronic adult periodontitis. It is the commonest type and is referred to as non-aggressive. The aggressive forms have been classified by Page et al. (1983) as follows:

Prepubertal: Affects children, usually involving the primary dentition soon after the teeth erupt and subsequently the permanent dentition. There is usually intercurrent infection and affected children have a defect in host response with defective polymorphonuclear and monocyte chemotaxis and adherence. Localised and generalised forms have been reported. May occur as part of other syndromes (e.g. Papillon-Lefèvre syndrome).

Juvenile: Occurs in teenagers with the age of onset between 11 and 15 years. When confined to permanent incisor and first molar teeth, it is referred to as localised juvenile periodontitis. If other teeth are involved, the condition is described as generalised. In the localised form, the lesions are frequently symmetrical producing a 'mirror-image' effect. As with prepubertal periodontitis, there may be impaired white cell function.

Rapidly progressive: Occurs in patients usually between the ages of 20 and 30 with severe and rapid bone loss.

Refractory: A type of periodontitis occurring in adults which progresses relentlessly to loss of the teeth in spite of all treatment. Some authorities deny the existence of refractory periodontitis attributing its progression to 'lousy treatment'.

ANUG-related: A form of periodontitis occurring in adults in which advancing bone loss is associated with acute necrotising ulcerative gingivitis. The diagnosis of this condition should include a strong suspicion that the patient may have AIDS.

AIDS-related: Very severe advanced periodontal disease is a feature of many patients with AIDS.

**161** The lower left central incisor looks abnormally long, especially in contrast to the lateral incisors which are in the process of erupting. However, this tooth does not exhibit recession which is by definition the apical movement of the gingival margin to the extent that root surface is exposed. What has happened in this case is that the gingival margin has matured to its adult level some 2–3 years earlier than usual. No treatment is required. As the child becomes older the mucogingival junction will move apically and the width of the attached gingiva will increase. It is possible that the underlying alveolar bone is thin or even absent (dehiscence) in which case true recession may occur in the future.

**162** The patient is Vietnamese. The stain was deliberately applied to enhance personal appearance. Cosmetic staining of teeth is fairly common in parts of the Far East. The method of application of the stain is complicated and varies from one community to another but the effect is a form of acid etching. This patient declined further attempts to remove the stain when scaling instruments failed. It is likely that rotating stones and/or burs would be required, followed by veneers or crowns.

**163** (a) (i) Inadequately fitting subgingival crown margin establishing a local plaque retentive factor. (ii) Retained subgingival cement following cementation. (iii) If the tooth is non-vital and root treated, then there may be a root crack retaining plaque .
(b) (i) Clinical and radiographic assessment. (ii) Removal of the subgingival irritant.
● Inadequate crown margin – replace with a well-fitting and polished provisional crown restoration, improve plaque control and replace the crown with a definitive restoration when the soft tissues have healed.
● Remove the subgingival cement and use an ultrasonic instrument to clean the subgingival area. Follow this with plaque control reinforcement.
● Reflect the gingival tissue to confirm the diagnosis and later extract the tooth when an appropriate provisional replacement has been constructed.

**164** (a) In standard smears of debris from ulcers in patients with ANUG it is usual to see: fusiform filamentous Gram-negative rods (ie spindle-shaped filaments with pointed ends), typical of *Fusobacterium* species; loosely coiled spirochaetes, probably *Treponema* species (but sometimes described in the older literature as *Borrelia vincentii.*); other, mainly Gram-negative bacteria, often seen as curved rods; polymorphonuclear leucocytes. This characteristic microscopic appearance has give rise to the expression 'fuso-spirochaetal complex' to describe the microbial flora associated with ANUG.
(b) The predominant micro-organisms reported by dark-field microscopy are: medium-sized spirochaetes (*Treponema* species, about 32% of total microscopic flora); motile, curved rods (probably *Selenomonas* species, about 6% of total microscopic flora).
(c) The predominant micro-organisms cultured from patients with ANUG are obligate anaerobes and include the following: *Prevotella intermedia* (formerly called *Bacteroides intermedius*, a black-pigmented, Gram-negative, anaerobic rod, comprising about 24% of the total cultivable flora); *Fusobacterium* species (obligately anaerobic, Gram-negative, fusiform rods, comprising about 3% of the total cultivable flora); a wide range of other bacteria, in smaller numbers, including streptococci, veillonellae and *Actinomyces* species.
(d) In addition to local debridement and scaling, improved oral hygiene and the use of antiseptic mouthwashes (such as chlorhexidine), systemic treatment with metronidazole is the drug of choice in most cases (e.g. 200mg three times per day for 3 days). This antimicrobial agent, originally developed for treatment of protozoal infections such as *Trichomonas* vaginitis, is highly effective against obligately anaerobic bacteria. Patients with ANUG can also be treated with penicillin.

**165** Mechanical cleaning in chronic gingivitis:

(i) Supra- and subgingival scaling with hand instruments.

(ii) Supra- and subgingival plaque removal with polishing instruments (brushes and rubber cup) and abrasive pastes.

(iii) Supra- and subgingival plaque and calculus removal by ultrasonic scaling and other oscillating devices.

(iv) Supra- and limited subgingival plaque removal by toothbrushes and interdental cleaning devices.

**166** (a) (i) Loss of bone support for the upper anterior teeth as a result of undiagnosed chronic adult periodontitis. (ii) Lack of posterior occlusal stability. (iii) Parafunctional clenching habit may have contributed to migration.

(b) (i) Periodontal treatment—involving oral hygiene instruction and removal of plaque retentive factors. Root planing and if necessary periodontal surgery if oral hygiene care justifies this. (ii) Provisional upper removable Michigan splint for night wear to protect against further migration. This could in addition be used to judge the appropriate vertical relation to be re-established. (iii) Orthodontic opinion to consider the feasibility of fixed appliance therapy to upright the migrated anterior teeth within the demonstrable vertical relation. Orthodontic treatment could only be contemplated in the event of periodontal health being established. (iv) Stabilisation of the posterior occlusion with removable, tooth-supported appliances.

**167** (a) The condition is hereditary gingival fibromatosis. This is an autosomal dominant condition that may be generalised or localised. The latter is more common and generally involves the maxillary tuberosities or retromolar pad and distolingual gingivae.

(b) The condition is often present from birth and therefore a careful history should aid the diagnosis. There may be a gradual increase in size during adulthood leading to false pocketing and interference with opposing teeth. If the latter occurs or secondary periodontal problems are associated, or perhaps the tissue is interfering with denture construction, surgical excision may be performed, although the condition sometimes returns. If symptom-free and there are no adverse periodontal complications, no treatment is indicated.

**168** The gingival condition has relapsed because of excess osseous investment of the lower incisors. This abnormality was first described by Alldritt. Normally, the alveolar bone margin is approximately 1·5mm apical to the enamel–cement junction. Where there is excess osseous investment, the bone margin may be close to, or even overlap, the enamel. The radiograph shows such a relationship between the teeth. In order to establish a normal relationship, labial and lingual flaps need to be raised and the bone carefully reduced to a correct level, at which stage the flaps are trimmed and apically repositioned.

**169** Antimicrobial action: Chlorhexidine is a cationic antiseptic and adsorbs to the negatively charged bacterial cell wall. At low concentrations, leakage of bacterial cytoplasmic contents occurs to cause bacteriostasis which is reversible, but if persistent cell death will occur. At high concentrations, chlorhexidine will precipitate bacterial cytoplasm and is bactericidal. Plaque inhibitory action: Chlorhexidine as a dication can adsorb to negatively charged receptors on pellicle-coated tooth surfaces, probably as a molecular monolayer. This locally adsorbed antiseptic provides a persistent bacteriostatic effect on micro-organisms which adhere to the tooth surface. This persistence of action on the surface, or substantivity, can last for 12-14 hours which supports the twice daily use of this antiseptic. Studies using low doses of chlorhexidine, applied only to tooth surfaces, revealed plaque inhibition equal in whole-mouth dosing to mouthrinsing. These data do not support therefore the oral depot slow -release mechanism as important in plaque inhibition.

Clinical uses: overall for the short-to-medium term control of the oral microflora and/or supragingival plaque, particularly when mechanical tooth cleaning methods are difficult or temporarily suspended.
(i) Adjunct to mechanical tooth cleaning in the early oral hygiene and therapy stages of periodontal treatment. (ii) Postoperatively in oral and periodontal surgery.
(iii) Patients with intermaxillary fixation. (iv)Postoperatively following root planing.
(v) Oral hygiene in physically and/or mentally handicapped patients. (vi) Oral hygiene in medically compromised individuals. (vii) Adjunct to oral hygiene and in the control of oral ulceration in the early phases of fixed and removable orthodontic appliance therapy. (viii) Management of recurrent minor aphthous ulceration. (ix) Management of oral candidal infections notably chronic atrophic candidiasis (denture sore mouth).
(x) Adjunctive use with fluoride in high-risk caries individuals.

**170** In order to minimise the risk of disease progression in such cases, it is essential that the patient is motivated to a very high standard of oral hygiene. Grade 1 defects with pockets deeper than 4mm may be successfully treated with an apically repositioned flap. Grade 2 defects are difficult to manage successfully because of the impossibility of achieving good plaque control. In these cases residual disease after treatment should be expected and minimised by frequent instrumentation of the furcation area. Root resection, hemisection or guided tissue regenerative techniques may be appropriate in some cases. Grade 3 (through and through) defects, if sufficiently large, can be treated by open curettage (apically repositioned flap) and subsequently cleaned with bottle brushes. Sometimes, additional interadicular bone may be removed (tunnel preparation) to faciliate this. Obviously such cases are endangered by excessive bone loss and susceptibility to caries attack.

**171** (a) GCF is a serum transudate when it emerges from healthy gingival sites. It passively moves across the junctional epithelium and is thought to carry with it all components normally found in serum. It also collects various products of host and bacterial cell metabolism, which collect in the local crevicular environment prior to appearing at the gingival margin. When the gingival tissues are inflamed or mechanically stimulated, it becomes a serum-like exudate.
(b) Other media which are under investigation for markers of disease activity are serum, saliva, venous blood and plaque.
(c) GCF is normally collected over a 30-second period or less. If collected over longer periods of time, the irritation to the junctional epithelium is thought to stimulate serum movement and the GCF collected loses its unique characteristics and becomes more serum-like in nature. It therefore loses its diagnostic potential.

**172** The division of inflammatory plaque-induced periodontal disease into initial, early and established lesions (gingivitis) and the advanced lesion (periodontitis) was suggested by Page as a means of understanding the timing of the complex changes which occur in the inflammatory process. This assumes the pre-existence of periodontal health and would be the sequence of events (up to the established lesion but not beyond it) occurring in experimental gingivitis when dental students, having achieved near-perfect gingival health, refrain from cleaning some or all of their teeth for 21 days. In all cases the gingivitis becomes apparent by this time (an established lesion). The initial and early lesions are not clinically detectable.

(a)  The initial lesion is characterised by:
- Vasculitis of the vessels subjacent to the junctional epithelium.
- Exudation of fluid into the gingival sulcus.
- Increased migration of leucocytes through the junctional epithelium and into the gingival sulcus.
- Presence of fibrin and serum proteins extravascularly.
- Change in superficial topography of junctional epithelium.
- Loss of perivascular collagen.

(b)  The early lesion is characterised by:
- Accentuation of the features of the initial lesion.
- Accumulation of lymphoid cells at the site of acute inflammation.
- Cytopathic changes in fibroblasts.
- Further loss of collagen fibre network.
- Beginning of proliferation of basal cells of junctional epithelium.

**173**  The established lesion in gingivitis, unlike the initial and early lesions, is clinically detectable and has the following features which may be seen in routine or specifically prepared histological sections:
- Persistence of acute inflammation.
- Predominance of plasma cells but no appreciable bone loss.
- Presence of extravascular immunoglobulins in connective tissue and junctional epithelium.
- Continued loss of connective tissue.
- Proliferation, apical migration and lateral extension of the junctional epithelium.
- Micro-ulceration of the junctional epithelium.
- Early pocket formation due to swelling of the gingiva.
- There is no significant bone loss.

**174**  (i) Persistence of features described for the established lesion. (ii) Extension of lesion into alveolar bone and periodontal ligament with significant bone loss. Osteoclasts may be seen adjacent to the bone. (iii) Continued loss of collagen subjacent to pocket with fibrosis at more distant sites. (iv) Formation of periodontal pockets with progressive loss of attachment. (v) Conversion of bone marrow distant from the lesion into fibrous connective tissue.

**175**  The brush is termed an interspace or interproximal brush. The purpose of the brush is to remove plaque from the embrasure area and as far interproximally as possible. Other interdental cleaning devices are 'bottle brushes', dental floss and tape, toothpicks and wood sticks. Interdental cleaning devices are required since most interdental sites are inaccessible to the mechanical influences of the conventional toothbrush. Despite the advantages of interdental cleaning devices as with toothbrushes they may cause damage to gingival tissues. Over-vigorous use may cause acute inflammation or frank ulceration of the gingivae. Frequent use, particularly of floss, may inflict chronic trauma to the epithelial attachment area and loss of attachment can occur. Wood sticks may break interdentally and be difficult to remove; the impacted material can swell to cause pain or act as a focus for infection.

**176**  (a)  (i) Pocket elimination or reduction for advanced pocketing, particularly around posterior teeth where a cosmetically acceptable clinical crown height is not so important.

(ii) Crown lengthening for teeth of short clinical crown height which are to be crowned or used as abutments. The ARF can be used with, or without removal of crestal alveolar bone.
(b) Comparison with gingivectomy: (i) Direct access to alveolar bone and infrabony pockets. (ii) Opportunity to preserve the full width of keratinised gingivae by placing it apically. (iii) Opportunity to deepen slightly the adjacent vestibular sulcus. (iv) Less healing by secondary intention (granulation).
(c) (i) Vertical relieving incisions are usually required and these may cross underlying root surfaces exposed by bony dehiscences or fenestrations, and if covered by thin mucosa, wound breakdown may occur. Oblique relieving incisions may expose crestal bone when the narrower marginal tissue is located apically on the wider alveolar base. (ii) Flap management can be demanding. Retaining and stabilising the flap in a more apical position requires careful placement of anchoring and marginal sutures and the periodontal dressing. (iii) Irregular underlying crestal bone contour and residual infrabony pockets can create either excess tissue coverage (e.g. in the case of a severe bony dehiscence), or exposed bone (usually interdental) and/or incomplete adaptation of the flap margin. (iv) Postoperative swelling and bruising are seen more frequently where extensive flap elevation has occurred. (v) ARF cannot be satisfactorily used where local anatomy prevents soft tissue apical repositioning e.g. on palatal surfaces and adjacent to prominent external oblique ridges with a shallow or non-existent sulcus.

**177** Diagnosis: localised juvenile periodontitis.
Treatment: (i) Any hopelessly involved teeth will have to be extracted. (ii) 2–3 week course of antibiotics (250 mg oxytetracycline 4 times daily) concurrent with root planing and surgery where necessary. (iii) Oral hygiene instruction and frequent maintenance recalls.

**178** Complications occurring within one week of gingivectomy could include:
(i) Loss of dressing. This may be due to failure to achieve good haemostasis following the surgery, too large a dressing being placed, the patient dislodging the dressing with injudicious chewing on hard food or injudicious brushing of the area. A useful way of securing periodontal dressings is to use a dental floss or tape ligature incorporated in the dressing immediately after placement and before it is completely set. The knot should be tied buccally and covered with a small extra piece of dressing to avoid annoyance to the patient.
(ii) Pain and swelling. This is usually due to postoperative infection and may require antibiotic therapy. Over-extension of the dressing may cause ulceration and pain.
(iii) Bleeding. In the absence of a bleeding diathesis, bleeding may be caused by postoperative infection of a loose dressing. It may also be caused by excessive physical exercise or alcohol.

**179** Calculus is calcified plaque. Both forms of calculus are similar chemically, consisting of approximately 80% inorganic and 20% organic matter. The inorganic matter is essentially calcium phosphate with traces of magnesium, fluoride and sodium. Bacterial plaque is common to both forms with the addition of material from saliva in the case of supragingival calculus and from gingival crevicular fluid in the subgingival variety.
   Supragingival calculus occurs on the clinical crowns of the teeth, is cream-coloured, relatively soft, not very adherent and occurs in greatest quantity opposite the ducts of the parotid and submandibular glands, i.e. on the buccal surfaces of the upper molars and the lingual surfaces of the lower incisors.
   Subgingival calculus forms on the root of the tooth within the pocket and may be incorporated within cementum. It is black or dark brown, very adherent, very hard and will become supragingival if exposed by gingival recession as in the illustration.

**180** (a) Acute herpetic gingivostomatitis.

(b) Hand, foot and mouth disease, herpangina.

(c) Malaise, anorexia, pyrexia. Anterior cervical and submandibular lymph nodes are enlarged and tender. Diffuse 'boggy' gingivitis with multiple vesicles which coalesce to form ulcers, usually scattered over oral mucosa, gingivae and tongue, but mainly anteriorly. (Herpangina ulcers are predominantly on the soft palate).

(d) (i) Reassure the parents; the disease is self-limiting in 7–10 days but they must be prepared for an irritable child and some loss of sleep for a few days! (ii) Give lots of fluids to prevent dehydration. (iii) Antipyretics and analgesics; paracetamol elixir. (iv) Consider specific antiviral agents; acyclovir is effective but only if given early in the natural history of the disease. Intravenous acyclovir is necessary for immunocompromised patients.

(v) Reduce secondary infection; in severe cases it is wise to prescribe systemic antibiotics to prevent secondary infection. Swabbing the mouth with 0.2% aqueous chlorhexidine also helps but young children will object. (vi)Topical relief of pain so that drinking is facilitated; lignocaine viscous or benzydamine hydrochloride. (vii) Rest; for very irritable children the use of promethazine will help to achieve sedation and sleep. (viii) Warn about the contagious nature of the disease and recurrent herpes labialis. (ix) Hot food will tend to cause discomfort so the consumption of cold food should be encouraged. (x) Arrange to see the child again in 3 to 5 days to confirm diagnosis, check effectiveness of treatment and ensure that the progression of the disease is satisfactory. If the child is dehydrated and acutely ill, then hospital admission for intravenous fluids, etc., may be required.

**181** The condition is primary herpetic gingivostomatitis. This presentation is a little unusual in that primary infection with the herpes simplex virus usually occurs in childhood and also in that there are no intra-oral vesicles or ulcers. Until recently some clinicians would have labelled this 'coccal gingivitis' or 'streptococcal gingivitis' on the dubious grounds that a swab of the mouth would grow cocci in culture. This is hardly surprising since cocci are the commonest oral commensals.

**182** The only precaution necessary in the case of patients who are taking monoamine-oxidase inhibitors and require a local anaesthetic is to avoid intravascular injection. Many dentists are under the mistaken impression that such patients and those who have hypertension should not be injected with the standard anaesthetic solution of 2% lignocaine with 1:80 000 adrenaline. This is, however, perfectly safe provided that an aspirating syringe technique is used and intravascular injection thereby avoided. Two per cent lignocaine with adrenaline gives more profound anaesthesia than any other solution and there is likely therefore to be less circulating adrenaline than would occur if a less potent anaesthesic agent were used and the patient's endogenous adrenaline liberated as a result of anxiety and discomfort. On the other hand, local anaesthetics containing noradrenaline as a vasoconstrictor should never be used as it has been shown to have caused death from hypertension.

**183** (a) This cannot be made from the radiograph. A vitality test is necessary and should the tooth be non-vital the diagnosis is a primary endodontic lesion with secondary periodontal involvement.

(b) (i) Endodontic treatment for 36 using a laterally condensed guttapercha root filling technique. (ii) Review of the periodontal healing. In this case, complete resolution of the periodontal lesion occurred following the endodontic treatment.

**184** Some powered scalers, especially the ultrasonic variety, must not be used in the vicinity of a person with certain types of cardiac pacemaker. Before the ultrasonic portion of this instrument is used, ensure there is no such person in the surgery. Powered scalers are used with a very light touch, there is therefore little or no tactile sensation for the operator and this, together with obscured vision due to the water spray, means that damage could be caused to the gingivae unless great care is taken. For the same reason it is not possible to use powered scalers to the full depth of pockets and completion of subgingival scaling must be with hand scalers. Excessive pressure or failure to keep the scaling tip on the move can cause damage to the tooth surface, especially cementum and dentine. Insufficient water coolant will cause overheating of the power-generating source, the tip and the tooth surface.

**185** In this case 25 and 36 have been extracted. 26 and 37 have both moved forward and tilted and 35 has over-erupted. As a result the distal enamel-cement junction of 35 is much higher than the mesial enamel-cement junction of 36. Nevertheless, the distance between the bone margin and the enamel–cement junction is the same in the case of both teeth and no pocketing is present.

**186** Mouthrinses offer the potential of delivering pharmacologically active substances around the mouth. In the management of plaque-associated gingival and periodontal diseases, the major potential of these rinses lies in the control of dental plaque. However, to date, effective rinses have contained agents which prevent plaque accumulation rather than remove accumulated plaque. Therefore this young lady will benefit only by using the rinse as part of a plaque control programme in which established supragingival plaque has either been removed professionally or by the patient using effective mechanical cleaning methods. As stated, the major limitation of rinses is their limited influence on established plaque and more importantly their total lack of action against subgingival plaque. Therefore, given the established nature of the patient's disease, unless there has been prior subgingival debridement, the mouthrinse (however effective against plaque accumulation) will provide no benefits to health. Other actual or perceived benefits of rinses in this condition would include short-term breath- and mouth-freshening; additionally some agents could assist stain removal from the teeth or inhibit the regrowth of supragingival calculus.

**187** (a) Enlarged, fibrous tuberosity.
(b) (i) Non-surgical management only. (ii) Gingivectomy. (iii) Wedge procedure. (iv) Box procedure.
(c) (i) Gingivectomy – buccal and palatal conventional bevelled incisions. Simple and quick technique, but leaves a large wound to heal by secondary intention. Haemorrhage may be a problem and, usually, there is a significant postoperative discomfort. (ii) Distal wedge – undermining incisions on buccal and palatal aspects of the tuberosity to create a wedge of tissue for removal which is wider at the bone base than orally. More technically demanding than gingivectomy because of limited access and angulation of incisions. May need to extend the incisions to develop undermining (or filleted) palatal and buccal flaps. Healing by primary intention can be achieved. Less postoperative discomfort than gingivectomy.
(iii) Distal box—a 3-sided pedicle flap with its base usually on the palatal aspect is prepared in order to lift the full-thickness tuberosity as if it were the lid of a box. The fibrous tissue on the underside of the flap is thinned by sharp dissection and the 'lid' is closed after trimming excess tissue from the flap margins. Again, access may be difficult and the procedure technically demanding.

**188** (a) 22 has a developmental groove. Examination during flap surgery showed that the groove extended to the apex.
(b) The prognosis is poor and the tooth should be extracted.

**189** The ulceration is due to excess pressure from the denture arising from resorption of the edentulous ridge. The denture pivots lingual to the lower canine teeth when the patient is biting. As an immediate measure the denture should be temporarily relined using a tissue conditioner. If necessary the denture may be eased lingual to 33 and relined with tissue conditioner. Until the ulcer has healed, it may be helpful to achieve plaque control by means of a chlorhexidine mouthwash. Steps should be taken to achieve periodontal health by improving oral and denture hygiene, removal of all deposits, and root planing where necessary. During this time the tissue conditioner should be replaced at intervals of 3 to 4 weeks. When the tissues are healthy a new denture which avoids coverage as much as possible of the gingival margins should be constructed. This should be checked for fit regularly and relined as necessary to compensate for ridge resorption.

**190** (a) Ankyloglossia ('tongue-tie').
(b) A mild degree of ankyloglossia is not usually associated with any problems, however, often the most significant is an interference with the normal oral self-cleansing mechanisms. Fraenal ulceration may occur and recession of the lingual gingivae if the fraenum is inserted high up between the lower central incisors. Ankyloglossia very rarely contributes to speech difficulties and only if very extreme.
(c) No treatment is usually required in infancy. A lingual frenectomy may be necessary in severe cases, usually to improve tongue mobility for oral self-cleansing.

**191** This is a common result of splinting mobile teeth without treating the associated periodontal disease. This woman's story was that 22 had become mobile some five years previously. Chronic periodontitis was almost certainly present and the mobility would have been caused by occlusal trauma from a tooth in the opposing jaw, probably as a result of parafunctional activity. She had consulted her dentist who splinted the 22 to 21 and 23 using composite resin and wire – the so-called A-splint. Thereafter the tooth was fixed and could not move under occlusal load which acted as a formidable co-destructional factor in the presence of active periodontal disease. This has led to exfoliation of the tooth with advanced bone loss now affecting also 21 and 23.
   The correct treatment for patients such as this is to treat the periodontitis as the first priority. When this is under control, occlusal examination will reveal the reason for the mobility which can usually be corrected by selective grinding.

**192** (a) (i) Inadequate proximal space for cleansing adjacent to the pontics.
(ii) Uncleansable concave fitting surfaces to the bridge pontics. (iii) Pontics constructed on a working cast altered to produce a 'socketed' effect for the pontics. This would have resulted in adverse tissue compression on cementation. (iv) Lack of oral hygiene instruction at the time of fitting the bridgework.
(b) (i) If possible re-use the existing bridge as a provisional. This will allow the restoration to act as a diagnostic appliance, both to correct the decementation problem and to modify to allow appropriate cleansing. The teeth will need to be re-prepared to establish good retention. The canine abutment particularly will need modification to ensure that the post core is of adequate length and the subsequent retaining crown can enclose tooth tissue. Following re-preparation, the bridge can be relined with a temporary crown and bridge resin to allow it to be re-used provisionally. (ii) Modify the proximal area between retaining crown and pon-

tics to allow the use of a proximal surface brush or, at the very least, a floss threader to carry dental tape between the abutments and pontics. (iii) Modify the fitting surface of the pontics to ensure minimal tissue contact and a convex cleansable fit surface. Polish the fit surface of the pontics. (iv) Modify the anterior guidance to prevent further decementation. If there is a parafunctional habit, then an occlusal appliance for night wear of Michigan design would be appropriate. (v) Reconstruct the bridge incorporating the design modifications once the soft tissue disease has resolved and the decementation problem is corrected.

**193** While it is true that many epidemiological surveys have shown that in children of both sexes there tends to be a transient increase in gingivitis at the time of puberty, it is rarely if ever possible to demonstrate the influence of the hormonal changes associated with puberty in the individual child. In this patient the causative factor of the gingivitis is plaque and instruction in plaque control and monitoring of progress is all the treatment she requires.

**194** The answers given below follow the recommendations given in the *British National Formulary* No. 25 (March 1993), based on the recommendations of a Working Party of the British Society of Antimicrobial Chemotherapy (*Lancet* 1992, **339**:1292).
(a) The normal recommendation for an adult patient, not allergic to penicillin, for a surgical procedure under local or no anaesthesia is: 3g single oral dose of amoxycillin, taken under supervision, one hour before the dental procedure.
(b) If the patient is allergic to penicillin, or has had penicillin more than once in the previous month, oral clindamycin should be prescribed (600mg taken under supervision 1 hour before the dental procedure). Clindamycin has replaced erythromycin as an alternative to penicillin, since erythromycin frequently causes nausea and vomiting. Until recently, clindamycin was not generally recommended for prophylaxis because of worries about possible side-effects including pseudomembranous colitis, but such effects do not appear to occur after a single oral dose.
(c) For patients undergoing general anaesthesia, who are not allergic to penicillin, the recommended prophylaxis is: intramuscular amoxycillin, 1g in a 2·5 ml 1% lignocaine hydrochloride just before induction plus 0·5 g by mouth 6 hours later; or, oral amoxycillin, 3g oral dose 4 hours before anaesthesia followed by a further 3g by mouth as soon as possible after the operation; or oral amoxycillin, 3g together with probenecid 1g orally 4 hours before operation. Patients who are allergic to penicillin, or who have had penicillin more than once in the previous month and require a general anaesthetic, should be treated as 'special risk' and are dealt with in section (c) of the answer to question 195.

**195** (a) It is recommended that special-risk patients, including those who have had a previous attack of endocarditis or who have prosthetic heart valves and require a general anaesthetic, or who are allergic to penicillin or have had penicillin more than once in the previous month, should be referred to hospital. Commonly the treatment will be planned after appropriate consultation between dental surgeons, cardiologists and anaesthetists, and is best carried out in an out-patient or in-patient hospital environment.
(b) For the non-penicillin-allergic patient, the recommended prophylactic regime is: 1g of amoxycillin intramuscularly in 2·5 ml of 1% lignocaine hydrochloride plus 120mg gentamycin intramuscularly just before induction; then 0·5g amoxycillin orally 6 hours later.
(c) For patients who are allergic to penicillin (or who have had penicillin more than once in the previous month), give either :
• Intravenous vancomycin 1g over at least 100 minutes, then intravenous gentamicin 120mg at induction or 15 minutes before the procedure.
• Intravenous teicoplanin 400mg plus gentamicin 120mg at induction or 15 minutes before the procedure.

- Intravenous clindamycin 300mg over at least 10 minutes at induction or 15 minutes before the procedure, then oral or intravenous clindamycin 150mg 6 hours later.
(d) When making a treatment plan for such complicated special-risk cases, every effort should be made to minimise the number of occasions when antibiotic prophylaxis is required. This may mean grouping operative procedures together so that as much as possible can be achieved while the patient is anaesthetised and covered by antibiotics in a controlled situation.

**196** There is evidence that early-onset periodontitis is associated with *Actinobacillus actinomycetemcomitans (Aa)* and that this micro-organism invades the gingival connective tissue; thus antimicrobial therapy should be used in these cases as an adjunct to surgical therapy. Aa is sensitive to tetracycline. In addition the drug is concentrated in crevicular fluid (5–10 fold the levels found in serum) and inhibits collagenases. The latter property may facilitate repair. Dosage of tetracycline in cases of early-onset periodontitis is 250mg x 4/day for 2–3 weeks.

Tetracyclines are broad-spectrum bacteriostatic antimicrobials. The main unwanted effect is disturbance of the gut flora leading to diarrhoea and superinfection of the mouth causing candidiasis. Staining of the teeth and bones is unlikely to be a problem in teenagers and young adults. Tetracyclines chelate with metallic ions, especially calcium. The chelate is poorly absorbed. Since calcium ions are present in many food substances, the patient should be advised to take the drugs half an hour before or after food. Tetracyclines can interact with the contraceptive pill causing 'pill failure'.

Such patients should be advised to use alternative contraceptive practice while taking the antimicrobial. In some patients, tetracyclines cause photosensitivity, thus they should avoid exposure to sunshine. Tetracyclines are contra-indicated in patients with renal and hepatic disease, since the drug is metabolised in the liver and excreted via the kidneys.

**197** (a) Cut test cavities without local anaesthetic.
(b) The most likely cause of the loss of vitality at such an early stage, is the presence of an invaginated odontome with pulpal communication, or an evaginated odontome which has been traumatically removed causing pulpal exposure. There are reports of teeth erupting with spontaneous exposures in the condition 'hypophosphatasemia', but serum phosphate levels in this patient were normal.

The non-vital pulp should be extirpated and the canals carefully cleaned prior to dressing with non-setting calcium hydroxide paste. The latter should be replaced at approximately 3-monthly intervals until a calcific barrier forms at the apex. At this stage the canals should be filled with guttapercha, taking care to achieve good apical and coronal seals.

**198** Migration of upper incisors: (i) In the case of this man loss of attachment due to chronic periodontitis has occurred. The loss of support for individual teeth coupled with the loss of crestal inter-radicular periodontal fibres can expose individual teeth to the influence of a variety of intrinsic and extrinsic forces, with the resultant effect that one or more teeth move forwards and on to a wider arc, resulting in spacing. Such forces may include the tongue and more particularly the lower lip behind the incisal edges of the upper incisor teeth, as well as occlusal forces from teeth in the opposing jaw. (ii) Habits such as thumb sucking or placing foreign objects behind the incisor teeth. (iii) Destruction of alveolar bone due to pathology in the area of the incisor teeth including, dental and developmental cysts, primary and secondary tumours. (iv) Supernumerary or supplemental teeth or odontomes in the midline. (v) Disease of bone enlarging the alveolar processes, e.g. acromegaly and Paget's disease.

**199** (i) The provision of a crown restoration in the presence of untreated chronic adult periodontitis. (ii) The crown restoration provision has contributed adversely to plaque retention in the presence of this untreated disease. (iii) Overcontouring the palatal surface of the left central incisor crown has led to the labial migration of this tooth. (iv) The labial migration has led to the loss of intercuspal contact with the crown restoration and subsequent over-eruption.

**200** (a) Localised juvenile periodontitis.
(b) There are currently three possible regimes which are in favour: co-amoxyclav alone, co-amoxyclav with metronidazole, or tetracycline alone. Co-amoxyclav is given as 250/125mg 3 times a day for 7 days either alone or with metronidazole 200mg 3 times a day for 7 days. Tetracycline is given as 250mg 4 times a day for 3 weeks.
(c) Checks should be made on whether the patient is pregnant (excludes all three drugs), allergic to penicillins (excludes co-amoxyclav), susceptible to candidal infections (excludes tetracycline). Any history of hepatic or renal impairment requires checking with the patient's physician before prescribing.

**201** Toothache tinctures were popular in the early years of this century. Although less commonly seen now, they are still available and no doubt many bottles still reside in domestic medicine cupboards. Their main constituent is phenol, varying in concentration in tinctures examined from 1% to 27%, mixed in a volatile solution usually containing ether, chloroform and alcohol. Oil of cloves and camphor are other common ingredients. They were intended to be applied to the exposed pulp of a carious tooth where it was hoped that the phenol would cause necrosis of the exposed nerve endings. If bottles are stored for a long time, the volatile ingredients will evaporate leaving almost pure phenol in the bottle. Patients sometimes apply the tincture to the gum when they have toothache, producing sloughing of the epithelium and a painful burn. As always with local self-medication, the clinician has to question the patient carefully to ascertain the original cause of the pain as well as to treat the damage caused by the chemical burn.

**202** The penicillins are the drugs most frequently implicated in anaphylactic reactions. Other drugs implicated, but to a much lesser extent, include aspirin and lignocaine. Signs and symptoms of an anaphylactic reaction include nausea, rashes, rhinitis, abdominal pain, wheezing, dyspnoea, laryngeal oedema, hypotension, collapse and cardiac arrest. These features are attributable to the massive release of histamine and other vasoactive peptides from mast cells. There are two priorities with regard to the management of these reactions: to maintain the airway and to restore blood pressure. Adrenaline 0·5ml 1:1000 is administered intramuscularly. This dose can be repeated every 5 minutes up to a maximum of 1·5ml. The drug is a potent vasoconstrictor and will restore blood pressure and reduce laryngeal oedema. Intravenous hydrocortisone 100mg should also be administered since it will stabilise mast cells and prevent further release of histamine. If the airway becomes compromised, oxygen should be administered. In the event of obstruction, a cricothyroid stab should be carried out with a large bore needle. Pulse and blood pressure must be monitored throughout this potentially life-threatening reaction.

**203** (a) Desquamative gingivitis.
(b) (i) Lichen planus. (ii) Drug-induced lichenoid reactions e.g. with propanolol or methyldopa. (iii) Menopause, related to hormonal changes. (iv) Cicatricial pemphigoid (benign mucous membrane pemphigoid). (v) Pemphigus. (vi) Psoriasis. (vii) Contact sensitivity with certain drugs, e.g. toothpastes or chlorhexidine mouthwash. (viii) Systemic or discoid lupus erythematosus.

(c) Cicatricial pemphigoid is a non-acantholytic condition, i.e. the cells themselves are not destroyed as such, but antibodies are directed against the epithelial basement membrane. The latter are predominantly of the IgG type and stain with immunofluorescence. There is also a tendency for subepithelial bullous formation, due to the site of antibody activity and epithelial separation.

**204** The unwanted effect of gingival overgrowth is associated with phenytoin, cyclosporin and the calcium-channel blockers. There is no unifying hypothesis which unites these three disparate compounds. However, various models have been suggested to explain this unwanted effect. In simple terms, drug-induced gingival overgrowth occurs as a result of an interaction between the drug or its metabolite with the gingival fibroblast. Inflammation appears to enhance this reaction and the net result is an increase in fibroblastic activity and subsequent collagen and protein synthesis. It has been suggested that gingival tissue contains two distinct populations of fibroblasts, designated high and low activity. High activity fibroblasts are characterised by increased protein and collagen synthesis; the converse applies to low activity fibroblasts. In any individual, the ratio of high activity to low activity cells is genetically determined. High activity cells appear to be more sensitive to the actions of the drug and inflammatory mediators.

An alternative explanation may be related to a drug-induced inhibition of collagenase production. The latter is an enzyme produced by fibroblasts which breaks down collagen. It is responsible for maintaining connective tissue homeostasis. Any inhibition of collagenase production could lead to excess connective tissue, and hence the appearance of gingival overgrowth.

**205** The gingival enlargement is caused by phenytoin – an anticonvulsant used in the management of epilepsy and other convulsive disorders. The enlarged gingival tissues are preventing adequate mechanical plaque control. Surgical excision is required to restore the gingival contour. Recurrence is a problem with patients on phenytoin therapy. This can be reduced considerably by the patient maintaining meticulous plaque control. Chlorhexidine mouthrinses, 0·2% w/v 10ml twice a day, are useful in helping to maintain good plaque control. Similarly, there is some evidence that folic acid mouthrinse (1mg/ml) 10ml twice a day can prevent the recurrence of phenytoin-induced gingival overgrowth. Many patients suffering from epilepsy and medicated with phenytoin are troubled with gingival problems. For these patients it is worthwhile discussing with their physicians a change in anticonvulsant therapy. Useful alternatives include carbamazepine and sodium valproate.

**206** (a) The causative micro-organisms are almost invariably endogenous, their most likely source being subgingival plaque.
(b) Local trauma or impaction of calculus following scaling in the soft tissue wall of the pocket are sometimes identified as significant factors.
(c) As with other purulent infections in the oral cavity, the microflora associated with lateral periodontal abscesses is usually mixed. The types of organisms commonly found include:
- Anaerobic Gram-negative rods or filaments, such as black-pigmented *Porphyromonas* or *Prevotella* species (formerly called *Bacteriodes*) and *Fusobacterium*.
- Oral streptococci and anaerobic cocci (such as *Peptostreptococcus* species).
- A variety of other bacteria, including *Actinomyces* species, *Capnocytophaga* species, and spirochaetes.
(d) Treatment is usually surgical, in order to achieve drainage of pus, and may necessitate tooth extraction.

If the patient has pyrexia or cellulitis, or if extraction has to be postponed until the acute infection has subsided, antibiotics should be prescribed. Penicillin, metronidazole and amoxycillin are often the drugs of choice.

**207** Xerostomia can be caused by a variety of conditions ranging through localised disorders of the salivary glands, certain types of systemic disease, radiotherapy and drug therapy. Local disorders of the salivary glands include Sjögren's syndrome, salivary calculi and certain neoplasia. Xerostomia is frequently associated with AIDS and diabetes mellitus. Radiotherapy to the head and neck often affects the parotid gland causing a marked reduction in salivary flow. Drugs commonly implicated in causing xerostomia include lithium salts, tricyclic antidepressants, $H_1$-receptor blockers (antihistamines), atrophine, antiparkinsonian drugs and phenothiazine derivatives.

Xerostomia renders the oral mucosa more susceptible to irritation and ulceration. There is an increased incidence of oral candidosis and caries, especially around the cervical margins. The wearing of dentures is made more difficult by xerostomia. Salivary substitutes are of value where there is minimal or no salivary flow. Examples include Saliva Orthana (mucin-based), Glandosane (methylcellulose-based) and Luborant (carboxymethylcellulose-based). Both Saliva Orthana and Luborant have a high pH which may help in the remineralisation of carious lesions. In the edentulous subject, a glycerin and lemon mixture may be of value, since there is not the risk of acid erosion associated with regular use of such a solution.

If there is still some residual salivary function, diabetic sweets and sugar-free chewing gum may promote some salivary flow. Pharmacological stimulation of the salivary glands can be achieved with cholinergic agonists such as bethanechol chloride, pilocarpine and pyridostigmine. Such drugs can only be used for a short period of time since they can have adverse effects on the gastrointestinal tract, cardiovascular and central nervous systems.

**208** Corticosteroids have a wide range of properties and affect many of the body's systems. The immediate problem is adrenocortical suppression. Supplementary corticosteroids suppress production of adrenocorticotrophic hormone with resultant atrophy of the adrenal cortex. When such patients are subjected to a stressful procedure—for example, periodontal surgery – their adrenal cortex is unable to produce sufficient cortisol to allow the body to cope with stress. The patient will therefore go into an adrenal crisis, characterised by hypotension and loss of consciousness. It is thus imperative that patients on systemic corticosteriods receive supplementary steroids prior to procedures which are likely to be stressful. The usual regime is to adminster such patients hydrocortisone hemisuccinate 100mg intramuscularly 30 minutes prior to the procedure. If the patient develops signs of adrenal insufficiency during the procedure, he should be given a further dose of hydrocortisone intravenously. Corticosteroids also suppress the immune system, are anti-inflammatory and can cause delayed wound healing. Therefore patients on these drugs show an increased propensity to infection. Prophylactic antibiotic cover may be required for these patients to prevent infection at the site of surgery.

**209** In formulating a treatment plan for an adult whose upper anterior teeth have drifted, there are three main facts which need to be determined before definite treatment can be planned. These are:
(i) Why did the teeth or tooth drift? In this case it would appear to be due to the tooth losing support because of periodontitis, thus making it more susceptible to movement following the application of occlusal forces, such as the forward posturing of the mandible on closure resulting from the occlusal prematurity. The condition has been aggravated by the

loss of control of the lower lip. Other factors which should be investigated include habits such as sucking the lower lip, thrusting the tongue between the teeth, holding a pen, nail-biting, bruxism, etc. (ii) Can the periodontal disease be eliminated? This depends upon the patient's compliance in oral hygiene, and the result obtained following scaling, root planing and, if necessary, flap surgery. (iii) Will it be possible to realign the tooth? This may be difficult if the space it previously occupied has been reduced by drifting of the other teeth, or if the lower incisors have over-erupted. It is important to obtain the advice of an orthodontist to ascertain the likely duration of orthodontic treatment and the type of appliance that will need to be used, with its obvious influence on the patient's appearance during treatment. The need for permanent retention will also have to be considered.

If all circumstances are favourable, a suitable treatment plan would be as follows:
(i) Thorough removal of all supra- and subgingival deposits by scaling, polishing and instruction in oral hygiene. (ii) Eliminate the occlusal interference by selective grinding. (iii) Assuming that the oral hygiene is excellent, after 3 months any areas which still bleed on probing should be root planed and appropriate periodontal treatment continued until the tissues are healthy. (iv) Only then should orthodontic treatment be carried out. The patient must be checked regularly during orthodontic treatment to ensure that oral hygiene remains at a high level and that periodontal health is maintained. (v) Regular maintenance.

It is vitally important that in such patients periodontal treatment should precede orthodontic treatment. This is because:
(i) Periodontal treatment is very patient-dependent and relies above all on the patient being able to maintain a very high standard of home care. This needs to be established early in treatment. (ii) It would be foolish to carry out extensive orthodontic treatment only to find later that the periodontal condition could not be resolved. Orthodontic treatment is predictable – periodontal treatment less so. (iii) Most importantly, orthodontic tooth movement acts in much the same way as occlusal trauma on a tooth with active periodontitis, as a co-destructive factor causing accelerated destruction of bone. It is not unknown for teeth to be lost during orthodontic movement when periodontitis has not first been controlled.

**210** (i) Developmental conditions such as 'hereditary gingival fibromatosis'.
(ii) Inflammatory enlargement, e.g. poor plaque control and chronic gingivitis, often aggravated by a lack of lip seal and/or mouth breathing. This may be oedematous, fibroedematous, or fibrous.
(iii) Drug-induced gingival overgrowth due to hydantoin (phenytoin or epanutin), cyclosporin-A, nifedipine and some other calcium-channel blocking drugs, or occasionally the oral contraceptive steroid. The drug-induced overgrowth is often a 'fibroepithelial hyperplasia' as opposed to purely fibrous tissue overgrowth.
(iv) Underlying haematological disorders, e.g. chronic benign neutropenia of childhood, acute monocytic leukaemia.
(v) Granulomatous disorders, e.g. Crohn's disease, sarcoidosis, orofacial granulomatosis (Melkersson-Rosenthal syndrome).
(vi) Wegener's granulomatosis.
(vii) Gingival fibromatosis associated with rare syndromes, e.g. Leband syndrome.

**211** Predisposing factors:
(i) Tooth position in the arch. Certain teeth and sites are more affected by the aetiological agents in gingival recession, e.g. trauma. (ii) Buccal or lingual placement of teeth in the arches or, in the case of upper multirooted teeth, wide separation of roots. Both factors are likely to be associated with reduced buccal and/or lingual alveolar bone coverage and buccal

placement in particular, although not exclusively, exposes the gingivae to chronic traumas. (iii) Developmentally absent, dehiscence thinned or fenestrated buccal or lingual alveolar plates.

Aetiological factors:

(i) Chronic trauma from toothcleaning habits. This is typically buccally sited and most marked in canine and premolar regions. Interdental recession may also be induced by plaque removal methods used in these sites. (ii) Habitual factitious injury from fingernails, foreign objects,etc. (iii) Chronic periodontal diseases. (iv)Acute gingival diseases, notably acute ulcerative gingivitis. (v) Periodontal and mucogingival surgery. (vi) Repeated root planing and scaling. (vii) Direct trauma from teeth in the opposing jaw in cases of Angle's Class II malocclusion when lower labial, upper palatal or both gingivae may be stripped.

Clinical implications of recession:

(i) Exposure of dentine to erosive and abrasive influences resulting in variable hard tissue loss. (ii) The same latter influences may cause dentine hypersensitivity. (iii) Exposure of dentine to aetiological agents in root caries. (iv) Poor aesthetics due to increased clinical crown length, differential dentine enamel colour or root discolouration from absorption by the dentine of extrinsic stains.

**212** This is a hyperplastic gingivitis associated with orofacial granulomatosis, which can be a localised entity, but may also represent the oral manifestations of sarcoidosis and Crohn's disease.

The aetiology of the localised form is uncertain, but may be related to some food or toothpaste intolerance. Biopsy is essential to confirm the diagnosis. Non-caseating, necrotising, epithelioid tubercle is the characteristic feature found in biopsy specimens.

It is important to screen such patients for sarcoidosis and Crohn's disease and if positive, refer them to the appropriate specialist. The localised lesion may resolve of its own accord. Corticosteroids, antimicrobial agents and surgery have all been used in the management of this condition. In some patients, food intolerance is important, and therefore switching to a low-allergen diet can produce a marked improvement. Patch testing is thus useful in these patients.

**213** Isolated abscess formation following scaling or root planing is usually due to bacteria being forced into the tissues during instrumentation. They may also follow displacement of a spicule of calculus into the soft tissue wall of a pocket.

However, two abscesses in a patient with a history of such lesions strongly suggests lowered tissue resistance to infection, commonly due to diabetes. In this case a urinary test carried out in the dental surgery was strongly positive for glucose and the patient was referred to her general medical practitioner for further investigation and treatment. After her diabetes has been stabilised, periodontal treatment can continue with every prospect of success. A history of recurrent lateral periodontal abscesses should always alert the clinician to the possibility that the patient may be a diabetic.

**214** (a)There is deposition of the acquired pellicle which rapidly coats exposed enamel surfaces. Pellicle is derived from saliva and is thought to be formed by selective adsorption of salivary components, particularly proteins. Interactions between acquired pellicle and the surface components of certain bacteria comprise one of the significant factors in early colonisation and plaque formation.

(b) Streptococci are conspicuous amongst the earliest colonisers, particularly *Streptococcus sanguis*. Most of the organisms found in early plaque are aerobic or facultatively anaerobic, and organisms such as *Neisseria* species and *Actinomyces viscosus* may be detected at an early stage.

(c)  As plaque develops the microflora becomes increasingly complex. Over a period of days, a greater variety of species can be found within the plaque so that by about 10 days there will be Gram-positive and Gram-negative cocci, rods and filaments present, as well as spirochaetes, representing a large variety of genera and species. In addition to becoming more complex, the environment within the plaque becomes increasingly reduced, thus allowing more obligately anaerobic organisms to become established. Such time-related changes are an example of 'bacterial succession'.

(d)  General characteristics of 'mature' dental plaque include: (i) the complexity of its microbial composition; (ii) the variety of bacterial species present; (iii) its variability from person to person and from site to site in the same mouth; (iv) accumulation of 'mature' plaque is associated with the development of gingivitis, which can be reversed by effective plaque control measures.

**215**  (i) Take a careful history to include investigation of the procedure and materials used in undertaking the endodontic treatment. This information may only be available from the dentist who carried out the work.

(ii) Clinical examination including radiographs of the affected site.

(iii) Surgical investigation of the area as soon as possible. This involves the removal of the sequestrum, which was due to the use of a paraformaldehyde-containing endodontic sealer expressed into the apical tissues.

Removal of the necrotic tissues in the periapical region will also be required with the placement of a retrograde restoration.

The patient should be warned that there will be some gingival recession following the procedure and that modification of the plaque control procedures will be necessary.

**216**  (a)  Reattachment is: 'The reunion of the fibrous periodontal attachment apparatus with a root surface on which a viable periodontal ligament exists'.

(b)  New attachment is: 'The formation of a new periodontal ligament and cementum, to a root surface that had a previously non-viable periodontal ligament (ie. a pathologically exposed root surface).'

(c)  Repair is: 'The replacement of necrotic/non-vital tissue with a fibrous tissue scar.'

(d)  Regeneration is: 'The biological process by which the architecture and function of a lost tissue is completely restored.'

(e)  'Guided tissue regeneration.'

**217**  (i) Make a detailed pocket chart for all teeth. (ii) Thorough sub- and supragingival scaling, polishing and instruction in oral hygiene. This may take 4–5 visits over 2–3 months to the hygienist who will carefully monitor progress using plaque and bleeding indices. This is sometimes called the initial or hygiene phase of treatment. (iii) The patient should be seen again after about 3 months and the oral hygiene checked using a plaque index – this may be partial or whole mouth. We will assume that the plaque control is excellent. All aspects of all teeth should be checked for bleeding on probing and the sites recorded. These are sites where active disease remains – perhaps because of remaining undetected calculus or cementum infected with bacteria or endotoxin. Root planing under local anaesthesia of these sites should be performed. (iv) The patient should be seen again after about 3 months during which time the hygienist will have made sure that the patient is well motivated and is maintaining the necessary high standard of home care. The sites which bleed will now be very few in number and in favourable circumstances if these are re-root planed active disease will be eliminated. (v) After a further 3 months any sites which remain active may be root planed as a closed procedure or via localised flaps.(vi) This should eliminate all active disease but the patient will need to be seen regularly and if breakdown occurs at any site, scaling and if necessary root planing will need to be carried out again.

**218** This is a lateral periodontal cyst. Although these are not common lesions, such developmental cysts occur most frequently in the canine and premolar region of the mandible. The correct treatment is to enucleate the cyst and subject it to histological examination, to exclude other possible diagnoses including an odontogenic keratocyst and adenomatoid odontogenic tumour.

**219** Where possible, try and avoid all drugs during pregnancy. The first trimester is the stage of organogenesis and hence the time of maximum teratogenicity. During the second and third trimesters, drugs are more likely to affect growth and function of normally formed tissues or organs.
   In dentistry, the following drugs should be avoided during pregnancy for the stated reasons:
(i) Aspirin and non-steroidal anti-inflammatory drugs – these can cause platelet impairment in the fetus and delay the onset of labour. If taken in the early stages of pregnancy, they can cause closure of the fetal ductus arteriosus *in utero* and persistent pulmonary hypertension.
(ii) Tetracyclines – increased risk of congenital malformations. From the fourth month of pregnancy onwards, tetracyclines are chelated with calcium and the chelate incorporated into developing teeth and bones. The drugs may also cause impairment of skeletal growth.
(iii) Metronidazole – animal studies suggest that this antimicrobial may be tetratogenic. Manufacturers recommend avoidance of the drug during pregnancy.

**220** Anticoagulant therapy is unlikely to affect the periodontal condition. Any bleeding from the gingivae is likely to be explained by the presence of plaque-induced gingivitis, unless the prothrombin time has been allowed to get too high. Patients should carry a card indicating the dose of anticoagulant and a record of prothrombin time tests. The latter is indicated by the international normalised ratio (INR). Depending on the reason for anticoagulant therapy, the dose is adjusted to keep the INR in the range 2.0–4.5. Scaling of teeth adjacent to inflamed gingivae should only be undertaken within a day or two of blood testing to ensure that the INR is within the prescribed range. If the INR is over 3.0, efforts should be made to reduce gingival inflammation by improving plaque control prior to sub-gingival scaling and then restricting scaling to a few teeth only per visit to reduce the risk of excessive bleeding.
   Periodontal surgery should only be undertaken following consultation with the patient's physician and/or haematologist. Some antibiotics potentiate the effects of warfarin and should therefore be prescribed only in liaison with the doctor.
   Analgesia in patients on anticoagulant therapy must always be by infiltration and never by block anaesthesia in order to minimise possibly dangerous haematoma formation.

**221** (a) The lesion is an abscess secondary to external resorption of the transplanted tooth. This has provided continuity between the pulp chamber and the periodontal tissues and the oral environment.
(b) (i) The removal of the buried tooth with minimal trauma is essential, since damage to periodontium and cementum will predispose to external root resorption.
(ii) There is good evidence that the insertion of a non-setting calcium hydroxide paste into the prepared root canal of a transplanted tooth within 14 days of transplantation will significantly reduce the incidence of resorption. It is suggested that this is related to the alkaline

environment that is created adjacent to any areas of root surface damage by the placement of the calcium hydroxide within the prepared root canal. Cementoblasts find an alkaline environment less favourable.

(c) 23 will have to be extracted and replaced in the short term by means of an immediate denture in acrylic resin. This can be replaced in due course by a denture of skeleton design in cobalt chromium. Althernatively, the patient may be considered suitable for an implant. If this is the case, after appropriate planning, 23 will have to be extracted with great care, and a decision made regarding the need for ridge augmentation by guided tissue regeneration (it is not uncommon for transplanted canines to exhibit bone dehiscence buccally). Given adequate bone support, the prognosis for an implant in a patient of this age with good oral hygiene would appear to be good, as long as the crown supported by the implant can be protected during both functional and, more particularly, parafunctional tooth contact. The aesthetic consequences of such protection must be very carefully considered in planning the most appropriate restoration.

**222**

| | *BPE* | *PSR* |
|---|---|---|
| <u>Code 3</u> | Treat by OHI, scaling and root planing, and reassess. | Detailed charting of affected sextant. If two or more sextants score 3, detailed charting of whole mouth, followed by appropriate treatment. |
| <u>Code 4</u> | Detailed charting of affected sextant(s) and appropriate radiographs of that sextant only, followed by appropriate treatment. | Full mouth charting and appropriate radiographs, followed by appropriate treatment. |

**223** (a) *Candida* species, usually *Candida albicans*. *Candida* is a yeast, one of the more common pathogenic fungi, which exists in a variety of forms including yeast cells (blastospores), pseudohyphae, true hyphae and chlamydospores.

(b) The condition is known by several names, including *Candida*-associated denture stomatitis, denture sore mouth, denture-induced stomatitis, chronic atrophic candidosis and chronic erythematous candidosis.

(c) (i) Direct smears: *Candida* hyphae or pseudohyphae can be demonstrated in smears from the mucosa or from the fitting surface of the denture.

(ii) Culture: *Candida* species can readily be cultured on Sabouraud's medium, but since the organism may be present in the healthy mouth, simple isolation is not necessarily diagnostic. Quantitative estimates of *Candida* colonisation of the mucosa and denture surfaces give a better indication of infection, and can be carried out by imprint cultures.

(iii) Biopsies are not generally indicated in this particular condition, but may be valuable in other forms of oral candidosis.

(iv) Titration of anti-*Candida* antibodies in serum is not generally used for diagnosis of *Candida*-associated denture stomatitis, but may be useful in other manifestations of oral candidosis.

(d) Both local and systemic factors may predispose to oral candidosis. Local factors include trauma, endogenous epithelial changes, quantitative or qualitative changes in saliva, and changes in the normal commensal flora of the mouth. Many different systemic factors may predispose to candidosis, including altered physiological, hormonal and nutritional states, and alterations to the body's immune mechanisms (i.e. immunocompromised patients).

(e) Treatment of *Candida*-associated denture stomatitis should include removal (and probably replacement) of the denture, improved denture and oral hygiene, and antifungal therapy. Antifungal agents that may be used include nystatin, amphotericin B, miconazole and fluconazole. The first three of these can be prescribed in the form of lozenges. The use of a general antiseptic mouthrinse, such as chlorhexidine, may also be valuable, but not in combination with a specific antifungal agent.

**224** (a) Cervicofacial actinomycosis.

(b) The most common aetiological agent is *Actinomyces israelii*, but other *Actinomyces* species, such as *A naeslundii, A meyeri* and *A odontolyticus*, are occasionally isolated. These species are usually found in mixed culture and a variety of other aerobic, facultative and anaerobic organisms may also be isolated including *Actinobacillus actinomycetemcomitans*.

(c) Macroscopically, look for small yellowish granules described as 'sulphur granules' in the pus. (*N.B.* Wherever possible, pus samples should be collected by aspiration into a syringe or during surgical incision and drainage; dry swabs are not appropriate). For microscopic examination, these sulphur granules should be washed, crushed and stained by Gram's method to reveal typical filamentous, Gram-positive branched rods, often in tangled masses. For isolation and identification of the causative organisms, crushed material from pus should be cultured anaerobically on blood agar plates for at least 7 days. *Actinomyces israelii* produces typical small, rough, 'molar tooth' type colonies.

(d) Cervicofacial actinomyces is an endogenous infection; the causative agents are commonly present in the mouth, particularly in dental plaque. The exact route by which the *Actinomyces* species reach the soft tissues is not always clear.

(e) Cervicofacial actinomycosis is the most common presentation, but thoracic, abdominal and pelvic forms of the disease also occur less frequently. Actinomycosis of the knuckles has occasionally been reported following a punch to the face, the assailants being infected from their adversary's teeth.

(f) Surgical drainage and debridement may be required, depending on the extent and duration of the infection. Actinomycosis often becomes chronic and this may be associated with extensive granulation tissue and fibrosis which inhibits the penetration of antimicrobial agents.

*Actinomyces* species are usually sensitive to penicillin and this is the antibiotic of choice in non-allergic patients. Either injectable or orally administered penicillin can be used, but treatment often needs to be continued for 6 weeks or more (up to 3 months in some cases). For patients who are allergic to penicillin, erythromycin or tetracycline are useful alternatives.

**225** (a) (i) Lateral periodontal cyst. (ii) Odontogenic keratocyst. (iii) Central giant cell granuloma. (iv) Odontogenic tumour.

(b) Enucleation and histopathological examination of the lesion.

This proved to be a calcifying epithelial odontogenic tumour (CEOT), or Pindborg tumour. This is a rare tumour, typically affecting the posterior body of the mandible in adults. Histological features are sheets or strands of epithelium in a connective tissue stroma. Foci of calcification are apparent on the radiograph and are a feature of mature tumours. These tumours are locally invasive and benign, but it is important to differentiate them histologically from poorly differentiated squamous cell carcinoma, which they can resemble. Following enucleation of the lesion, the patient has been free of recurrence for 4 years.

# Index

Numbers refer to question and answer numbers.